give me a
baby

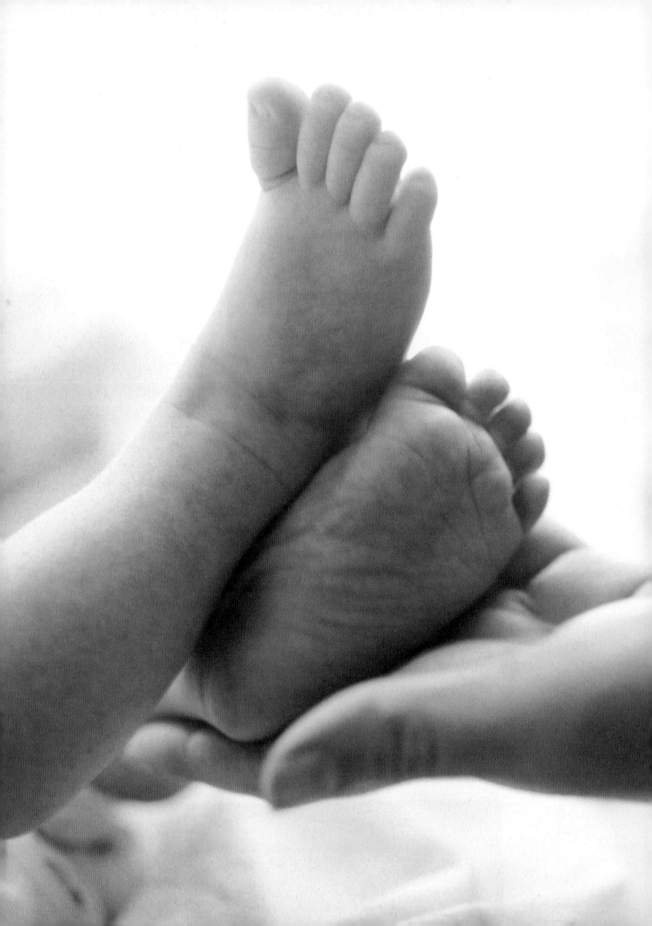

make me a

baby

Dr Simon Atkins

ACTIVE

This book is published to accompany the television series, *Make Me a Baby*, produced by Mentorn and first transmitted on BBC3.
Television series © Mentorn 2007
Executive Producer: Liesel Evans
Producer: Jennifer Gilroy

Educational Publishers LLP trading as BBC Active
Edinburgh Gate
Harlow
Essex CM20 2JE
England

ISBN 978-1-4066-1399-5
With thanks to Liesel Evans, Jennifer Gilroy and David Leach.

Commissioned by Emma Shackleton
Project Edited by Helena Caldon
Designed by Annette Peppis
Illustrations by Alan and Emily Burton
Picture researcher: Jeanette Payne
Production Controller: Man Fai Lau

Printed and bound by Graficas Estella, Spain

The Publisher's policy is to use paper manufactured from sustainable forests.

Contents

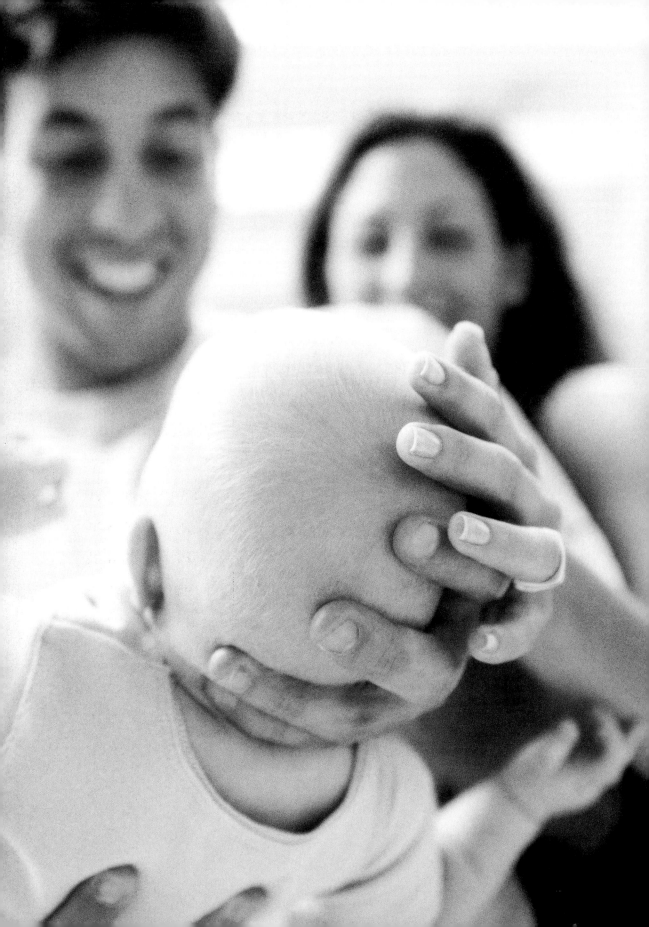

Introduction

People have been making babies ever since Adam and Eve first realized they were naked and that pruning the plants in the Garden of Eden wasn't the most fun you could have with your clothes off. And there seems to come a time in most couple's lives when they decide it's their turn to have a bash at starting a family.

For many couples there's no great game plan to conceiving, it's just a matter of getting down to business and hoping that they get it right. And there's nothing wrong with that approach – it often pays off in the end and they will probably have lots of fun along the way. However, other couples might choose to take another route. Their aim might be to plan conception in order to maximize the chances that the baby will pop out in the summer time (when the weather's just right for pushing a pram around or being off work), or so that its date of birth makes it the oldest child in its school year.

However, most of us are less demanding than this. We're just happy with a boy or a girl, an August or a September baby, but we are similar in that we probably still want a reasonably quick return for our efforts. And that's where this book comes in.

Make Me a Baby accompanies the groundbreaking BBC television series called… *Make Me a Baby*, in which we followed 100 couples from all over the United Kingdom through the trials and tribulations of trying to conceive and then, if successful, through their pregnancies and childbirth.

It was an amazing experience to learn from these couples the myths they had heard about various approaches to conception, especially those that would supposedly help them to achieve their 'baby of choice'. There seems to be a startling amount of misguided advice out there in books, magazines, websites – and often from so-called 'experts'. These gurus of conception recommend specific diets to follow, sexual positions to adopt, as well as the optimum frequency and timing of intercourse to ensure you get that longed-for boy, girl, or child genius. At best it's confusing and at worst, completely misleading. So it's not surprising that many of our couples were left scratching their heads about what to believe.

Both in this book and in the series, we wanted to cut through this fog of bewildering nonsense and instead highlight the latest scientific facts known about the often emotional subject of conception. So here I aim to provide sensible tips on how to maximize your chances of success by staying fit and healthy so that your eggs and sperm are too, and to convince you of the detrimental effect that extreme weight conditions and poor diet can have on your reproductive ability. For example, do vitamin supplements actually help fertility? And how much benefit will you get from ditching the fags and cutting down on the booze?

Of course, this is not to forget the most crucial aspect of making a baby – sex. Here you will find advice on what is the optimum time of the month to try and conceive, how often you should be having sex at that time so there's enough of his sperm available to do the job, and whether any sexual positions you can contort yourselves into can genuinely improve your chances of those sperm reaching an egg.

So once you've covered all this and the research has paid off, the rest of the book will take you right through the three trimesters of pregnancy, covering the dos and don'ts of each period separately. In addition, these chapters will explain how your baby is developing during each of these stages, what effect this will have on an expectant mother (and any warning signs to look out for for potential problems), and the corresponding check-ups that your doctor or midwife will want you to attend to ensure that everything's going smoothly.

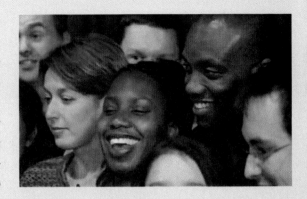

There's also more general advice along the way to help prepare you for your new life as parents; such as what you'll need to buy to kit out your little sprog ready for it's arrival and what you need to pack in your hospital bag for the big day itself.

And, of course, there's everything you could want to know (and possibly more) about what to expect from labour and birth, and the all-important options available to you for pain relief and safe delivery of your baby. Then, when you've got through all of this, there are some helpful tips and advice about bringing baby home and how you and your partner can prevent this life-changing event from creating too much chaos!

The journey from conception to the arrival of your baby is a magical one, which can be full of twists and turns and can involve some choppy waters along the way, but with good preparation, advice and support it can also be plain sailing. At the end of this adventure you will be rewarded with a very special gift; one that will bring you more ups and downs for the rest of your life – but it's worth it! So all it leaves me to say now is, read on and good luck as you make your baby.

Dr Simon Atkins

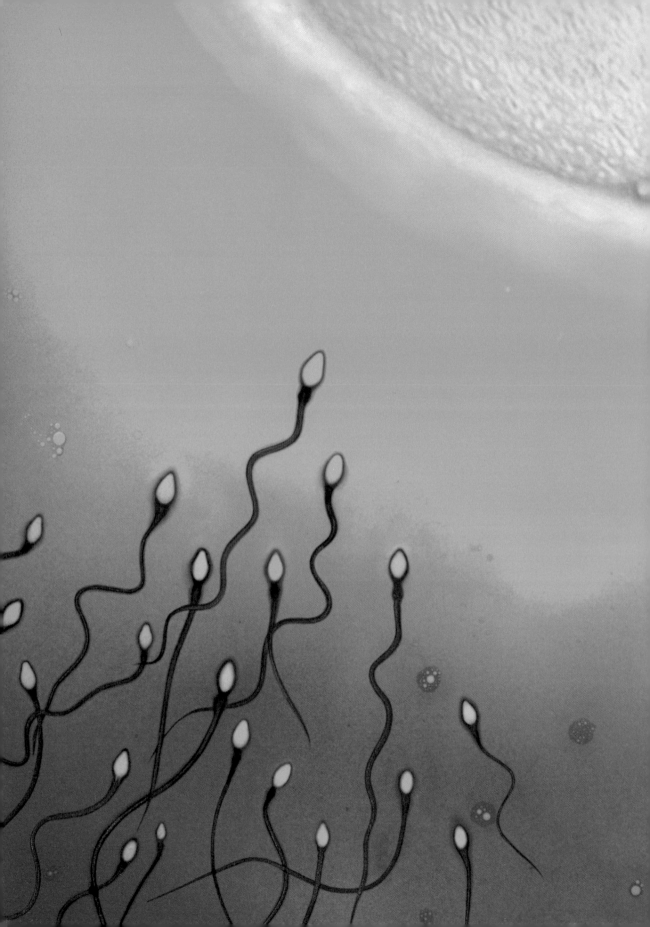

chapter 1

Conception

The story of how a sperm battles its way towards an egg to make a baby is one that is more action-packed than any of the biggest Hollywood blockbusters. There's more danger than Indiana Jones ever had to face, more challenges than in all of the Harry Potter movies, a higher body count than in *Saving Private Ryan*, and the principal characters do more to safeguard the future of the human race than every one of the six James Bonds put together – even with the help of their gadgets and their girls.

To would-be parents it appears that the journey to conception begins in a number of possible ways: from the planned attempt to hear the patter of tiny feet or to extend an existing family, to the failure to roll on a condom in the heat of the moment or to remember to pop a contraceptive pill. However, the story of conception actually began months or even years earlier in the couples' reproductive organs, at the time when eggs and sperm were first made.

The science bit

Reproduction is, of course, vital in order to keep our species going; it allows genes to be passed on to future generations. These genes are made up of massive molecules of a protein called DNA (deoxyribonucleic acid), which itself is made up of four smaller building blocks called amino acids.

These amino acids – called adenine (A), cytosine (C), guanine (G) and thymine (T) – are arranged in varying, but specific, orders in different genes, e.g. ACGTAGTATC in one and CTGTGCATCG in another (though the sequence is much, much longer for each). These sequences form a code which is translated by special molecules in our cells into the proteins which make up our bodies. As a result, we have a gene which specifically produces heart muscle thanks to its code, another for teeth, another for eye colour, and so on until a whole human has been made.

We each have a set of our genes in every cell in our bodies, contained in the central part of the cell: its nucleus. They don't randomly hang around in the nucleus but are packaged together in groups in chromosomes. Each parent passes on half of their chromosomes and therefore half their genes to their offspring in either their eggs or sperm. This mixing of genes from both parents (rather than all genes coming from just one) reduces the chances of defective or malfunctioning genes being passed on and, likewise, increases the chances of passing on any 'good' genes.

In the human body we have a total of 46 pairs of chromosomes, including two which are called the 'X' and 'Y' chromosomes. These chromosomes determine the sex of the baby: baby girls have two X chromosomes and baby boys have one X and one Y. The woman always passes on her X chromosome in her egg, whereas her partner can pass on either an X or a Y chromosome in his sperm.

His and her's
Sperm

Human sperm develop in men after puberty (which usually occurs during the early teenage years) in the testes (or testicles), which hang down outside the body in a sac called the scrotum. There is a practical reason

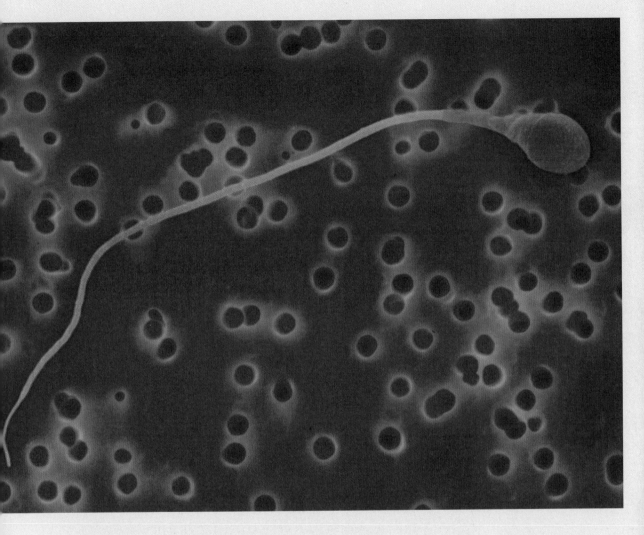

for this location, in that it ensures that the testes are kept a degree or two cooler than the organs inside the body and so at the optimum temperature for sperm development. This process takes around 70 days from start to finish and is repeated continuously throughout a man's life. However, the quality and quantity of sperm does begin to decline as a man gets older.

The mission for these sperm, of course, is to seek out the egg in the woman in order to fertilize it (see page 19). The structure of a sperm, therefore, is designed to maximize its chances of success in its quest. Each sperm cell has a tail to propel it forwards toward the egg, and also a head which contains all of the genetic material and which also provides the necessary apparatus for burrowing into the egg once it encounters it.

A normal, healthy-looking sperm cell.

Eggs

In contrast to men (whose sex cells develop rather later in life), a woman is born with all the eggs she will ever need already inside each of her ovaries. By the time a girl reaches puberty (again, probably in her early teenage years), she will have around 400,000 immature eggs ready and waiting to be released.

Unlike most mammals, who only become fertile and produce eggs at certain times of the year, humans produce just one egg each month as part of what is known as the 28-day menstrual cycle (see diagram below). This process is controlled by hormones that are released from the pituitary gland in the brain and has two main phases: the follicular phase and the luteal phase.

The follicular phase

On day one of the menstrual cycle the follicular phase begins, causing the ovaries to produce a number of tiny follicles. Between days six and eight, one of these follicles will produce an egg. On day 14 , ovulation occurs: the follicle enlarges and the egg is released into the fallopian tube. Some women actually feel this happening and experience what is called a 'mittelschmerz', or mid-cycle pain. At this time, body temperature will also rise by around half a degree centigrade.

A regular 28-day menstrual cycle will follow the pattern shown in this diagram.

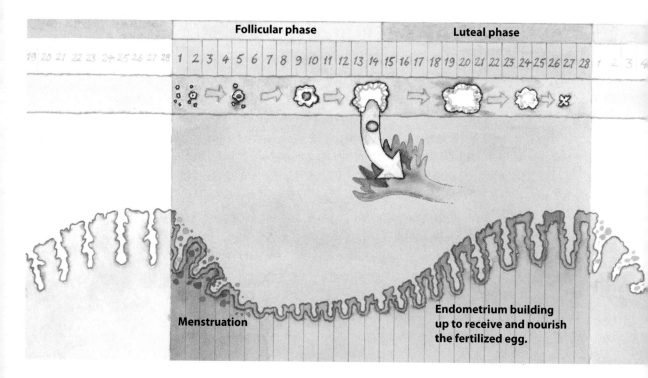

Follicular phase

Luteal phase

19 20 21 22 23 24 25 26 27 28 | 1 2 3 4 5 6 7 8 9 10 11 12 13 14 15 16 17 18 19 20 21 22 23 24 25 26 27 28 | 1 2 3 4

Menstruation

Endometrium building up to receive and nourish the fertilized egg.

The luteal phase

After ovulation comes the luteal phase, which occurs between days 15 and 28. This begins when the structure of the follicle changes and it becomes what's known as the 'corpus luteum' and produces high levels of a hormone called progesterone, which thickens the endometrium (the lining of the uterus). If fertilization has occurred by day 24, then the corpus luteum will go on operating to help the pregnancy continue by remaining active and producing progesterone. If however there has been no fertilization, the follicle shrivels up and triggers the start of the woman's period. Another cycle then begins, but this time in the other ovary.

In women whose periods do not fall into the textbook 28-day pattern, it is the length of the first follicular phase which tends to vary, while the luteal phase is pretty much fixed at 14 days.

> Eggs are much larger than sperm, and in laboratories they can be seen with the naked eye. They not only contain 23 chromosomes like a sperm, but they are also packed with energy-making cell components, called mitochondria, as well as nutrition for the embryo when it is first formed.

The journey begins

The process of getting these two cells together to create a new life begins with ejaculation. Up until this point the sperm have been holed up in the epididymis, where they've been stored for around two and a half months. But this cosy existence is abruptly interrupted when the contraction of the vas deferens (see diagram on page 17) unceremoniously propels them from their home during a process called emission. Once emission occurs full ejaculation is inevitable, as the man has reached what is often termed the 'point of no return'.

The sperm then whizz through the so-called ejaculation ducts. As they travel they are mixed with various nourishing and protective secretions from the seminal vesicles and the prostate gland, before rhythmical contractions shoot them out through the urethra (the tube which runs down the centre of the penis). All this activity occurs as part of the male orgasm, which usually lasts around 17 seconds or, if he's lucky, up to a minute.

Follow the dots for the route taken by sperm from testes to vagina during ejaculation.

The volume and the number of sperm ejaculated varies greatly from man to man and is affected by a number of factors – including the length of time since the last ejaculation. However, most men can expect to dispatch at least 40 million sperm.

Once ejaculated, the first and most crucial challenge for the sperm is simply to stay inside the vagina. And, to be honest, they're not very good at it. It is believed that millions of sperm trickle out of the vagina not long after ejaculation (in a process glamorously called flowback), and that within 30 minutes there's about 1 per cent of them left inside to carry on the journey.

Those that do manage to hang on in there have by no means made it. In fact, their troubles have only just begun.

Dodging the obstacles to the uterus

Humans have exceptionally good immune systems that can protect their bodies against invading micro-organisms – and invasions don't come much bigger than the millions of tiny sperm contained in a 5ml glob of ejaculated semen. So it's no surprise that the woman's body will attempt to get rid of these invading sperm in a variety of ways.

Acid attack

The first weapon the female body throws at the sperm is acid. Not by the bucket load, obviously, but the vagina is reasonably acidic (with a pH level of less than five) in order to comfortably see off many of the bugs that cause sexually transmitted infections. However, this acidity can also be potentially damaging to sperm.

Neutrophils

In addition to this acid attack, once the sperm have arrived in the vagina it doesn't take long before the woman's immune system has been sufficiently stimulated to cause white, infection-fighting blood cells called neutrophils to hurtle towards the area. These neutrophils attack and swallow up sperm during a process termed phagocytosis, which causes further depletion in the number of sperm.

This battle might sound a bit one-sided, however, sperm also have a few tricks up their sleeves to protect themselves. For a start they are deposited right at the top of the vagina, just a short swim from the cervix and relative safety.

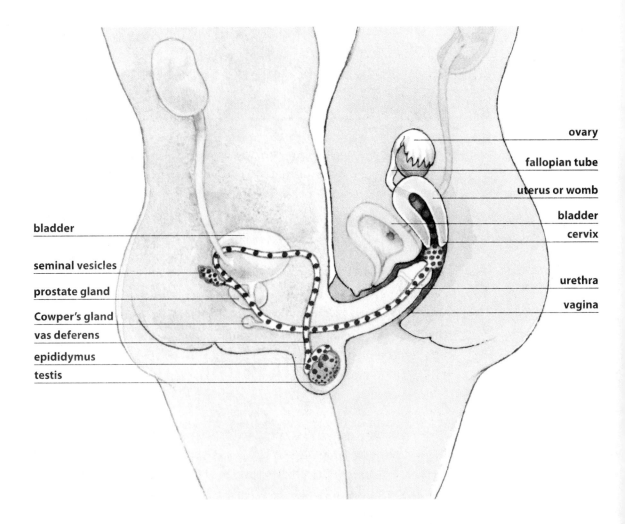

ovary

fallopian tube

uterus or womb

bladder

cervix

urethra

vagina

bladder

seminal vesicles

prostate gland

Cowper's gland

vas deferens

epididymus

testis

Secondly, each sperm is surrounded by a gel (made from some of the constituents of semen), which forms around them soon after ejaculation. This gel offers protection from the woman's immune system for up to one hour, neutralizes the acidity inside the vagina and holds the sperm close to the cervix.

Mucus plug

The only major obstacle left for the sperm in their bid to swim out of the vagina and into the womb is the plug of mucus in the cervix. Normal sperm have a good chance of advancing through this plug, but the mucus acts as a quality control and filters out the dud, odd-shaped or poorly swimming sperm. So by this point only a few thousand of the sperm that were initially ejaculated will make it through into the uterus.

Passing through the cervix is no picnic for the sperm, as it also has its own defences. However, it does offer help to the strongest survivors in the form of what amounts to microscopic swimming lanes. These lanes are created by threads of protein that run through the mucus and allow the sperm to swim in relatively straight lines through the centre of the cervix, thus avoiding the neutrophils that tend to hang around at the edges.

Moving on in

Sometimes sperm will hover in the cervix for up to five days, but most will immediately embark on the next step of the journey through the womb. At an average swimming speed of 5mm per minute this could take less than ten minutes. There's also good evidence to show that these swimmers are helped on their way by muscular contractions in the wall of the uterus, which help to waft the sperm upwards. However, there are more defences here too, and with most of their protective gel gone by this stage the sperm are now a lot more vulnerable to attacks by white blood cells.

The uterotubal junction is the gateway from the womb to the fallopian tubes. It's a bit tight: in fact, it makes the idea of a camel going through the eye of the needle completely plausible, being little more than a tight squeeze. Not only is the junction extremely narrow, but it is blocked by yet more mucus – the female reproductive tract has more of this stuff than a snotty toddler – and it can be completely compressed at times by the blood vessels around it.

With all these defences you'd think that the last thing the reproductive organs were designed for was reproduction. But there is some hope, and this comes in the form of specialized protein molecules which seem to be able to bind with each sperm and chaperone them through the uterotubal junction.

Once they have arrived in the fallopian tubes the sperm are virtually home and dry. The tubes are a spermy Shangri-La – not only is there an absence of defence mechanisms to battle against, but the tubes also act as reservoirs which protect the fertility of the sperm until ovulation. Here the sperm are fixed to the walls of the tubes until they are ready for the final stage of their journey – the assault on the egg.

The final hurdles

The last push to fertilization involves two different processes, which (to continue the military metaphor) turn the sperm into live ammunition capable of not only hitting their target, but of fertilizing it too.

These processes are called capacitation (during which the sperm is primed so it is ready to penetrate the surface of the egg) and hyperactivation (which changes the way in which the sperm's tail beats, thereby allowing it to swim more vigorously).

Capacitation begins the proceedings by causing biochemical changes in the head of the sperm to enable it to penetrate the surface of the egg. Hyperactivation then enables the sperm to weave in and out of the ridges and troughs that make up the lining of the fallopian tubes, turning the final leg of the sperm's journey into a maze.

The egg does, however, try to help the surviving sperm to reach their prize by using two forms of attraction. Firstly, it's warmer around the egg than it is in the tubes and this temperature difference guides the sperm towards their target, rather like heat-seeking missiles. And, secondly, chemicals released by the egg also seem to play a part by encouraging the sperm to turn towards it and by stimulating the tail to beat in such a way that the sperm can navigate the maze as easily as possible.

Reaching the journey's end

So, finally, the sperm are within touching distance of the egg and are able to complete the ultimate stage of their mission, and the one that they have been primed for.

Here the obstacles are removed at last. When a sperm comes into contact with the egg, a reaction occurs in the acrosome (the outer coating on the sperm's head) to allow it to pass through the outer layers of the egg – the rather wonderfully named corona radiata and zona pellucida.

Once one sperm has entered, electrical changes occur in the cell membrane of the egg to prevent more following it. The sperm then loses its tail and its nucleus fuses with the nucleus of the ovum to form a zygote – the first stage in a baby's development. After 36 hours this new cell divides and begins its journey down the fallopian tubes to the lining of the uterus, where it can implant and begin to form the placenta.

Meanwhile, the other poor sperm who have battled hard to reach the egg and endured all the trials and tribulations that the female reproductive tract has unleashed upon them, but have failed to reach their target, are either gobbled up by white blood cells in the fallopian tubes or expelled into the abdominal cavity to meet the same grizzly end.

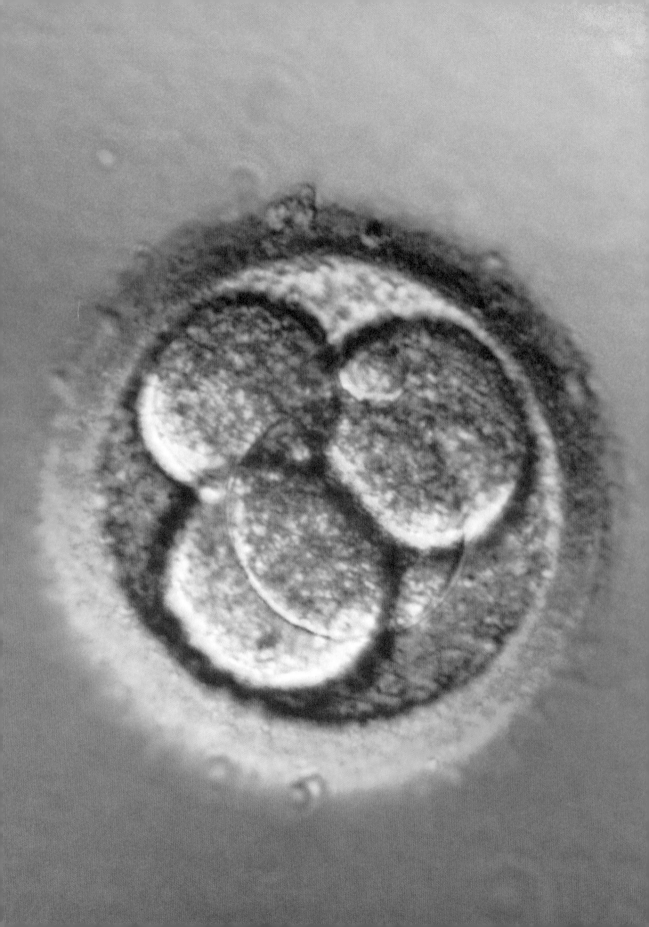

The conception gamble

Well, that's the science of conception which makes the whole breeding process sound a bit tricky. In fact, there are rumours which suggest that as a species our fertile days are over. Allegedly this is because oestrogen in our tap water is morphing men into their mothers; laptops are boiling their balls and even mobile phones have been implicated in a reduction in sperm counts (although personally I put mine to my ear).

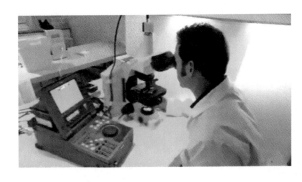

The quality of sperm in a semen sample can be analyzed using a microscope.

So with all that in mind, what are your chances of becoming pregnant? Well, actually, it's likely to be a pretty good 85 per cent in the first year of trying, which is encouraging. Unfortunately, though, one in six couples will eventually need to seek medical help in order to conceive because of problems with either their eggs, sperm or their reproductive plumbing. But for the rest it's just a matter of try, try and try again until your eggs and sperm get it together.

However, there are a number of factors that can help you maximize your chances of conceiving. Conception, like football, is a game of two halves – the chances of having a baby significantly increase if you both take the process seriously. You each need to look after your health, avoid bad habits that can affect your reproductive organs and, obviously, have a fair amount of sex.

So in this part of the chapter, we'll take a look at things that can prevent you both being match fit (to really milk the football metaphor…), as well as looking at when you should be having sex and how often you should be doing it.

Male fertility

Obviously you only need one sperm to reach an egg in order to make a baby but, as we've seen, the journey they have to make to get there will wipe out millions of them before they've even got close. So a man's main qualification for successful conception is that he has a decent number of sperm in each ejaculation, thereby increasing the possibility that some will get through.

These sperm also need to be pretty normal looking and good at swimming; you can have millions of sperm but if they are all abnormally shaped and only swim in circles, your chances of one of them reaching an egg are probably as poor as if you had hardly any sperm at all. So in the baby game, it's a question of quality as well as quantity.

This is what an embryo looks like under a microscope during early cell division.

SPERM COUNT

The World Health Organization has produced a range of normal values for semen, which suggest a minimum standard at which sperm are fit for fertilization (see below). If your levels match up to these then your chances of being able to do the business are pretty high. But even a man with a sperm concentration of less than 5 million sperm per millilitre still has a 19 per cent chance of fathering a child, so a lower sperm count need not always be the end of the world.

Volume	2ml
Concentration	> 20 million per ml
Motility (movement)	> 50 per cent moving forward
Morphology (shape)	> 15 per cent normal
Alive	> 50 per cent

Lifestyle factors affecting sperm

There's a good reason why doctors seem to go on about losing weight, keeping fit, eating a healthy, balanced diet, only drinking alcohol in moderation and never letting a lit cigarette touch your lips. It's because it's good advice – not only for the general health and wellbeing of your body, but also for your sperm. All of these factors can influence sperm production, along with a few other interesting ones that might seem less obvious.

Weight

In 2004 a Danish study showed that being both overweight and under weight can affect a man's sperm count. They looked at sperm samples from over 1500 young army recruits and found that sperm counts and sperm concentration were 28 per cent and 36 per cent lower, respectively, in underweight men (those with a body mass index of under 20) and 22 per cent and 24 per cent lower in the overweight group (whose BMI was greater than 25).

This result is believed to be due to the fact that men with high levels of body fat have less of the male hormone testosterone in their bodies (because the fat cells turn it into the female hormone oestrogen), and less testosterone means less stimulation of the testes to produce sperm. As for the underweight group,

It will come as no great surprise that if you both look after yourselves and have healthy and active lifestyles, you will greatly improve your chances of conceiving.

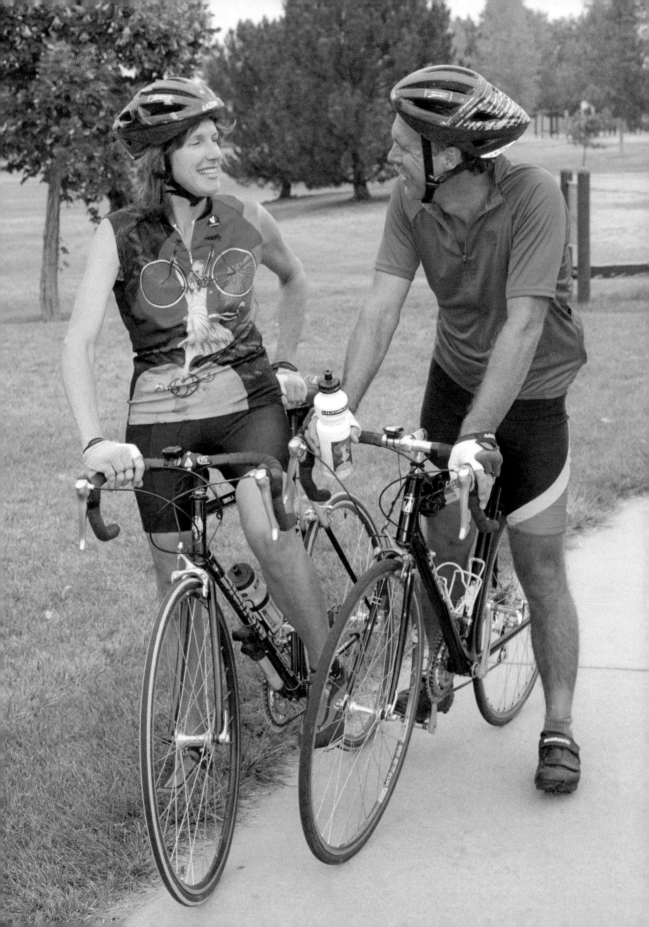

the researchers speculated that poorer nutrition or general health problems may well contribute to their lower counts.

So the bottom line is: if you want a decent sperm count, eat well to reach a healthy weight; and cut down on fatty foods if you're on the plump side.

Smoking

Surprise, surprise, smoking is not good for your sperm! A study published in 2007 looked at 2562 men who each provided semen samples and answered a questionnaire about lifestyle and factors related to health. The researchers found that the heavy smokers in this group had a 19 per cent lower sperm concentration than the non-smokers and that smoking also reduced testosterone levels. Other studies have also found that smokers have more abnormal, less mobile sperm, and it can particularly affect the sperm's tails – meaning that they have little chance of going anywhere fast!

As with other parts of your body, smoking and drinking will do your fertility no favours either.

And it isn't just tobacco that can have an effect on fertility: studies have also shown that smoking marijuana regularly makes sperm swim too fast, so they run out of steam long before they ever get close enough to reach an egg.

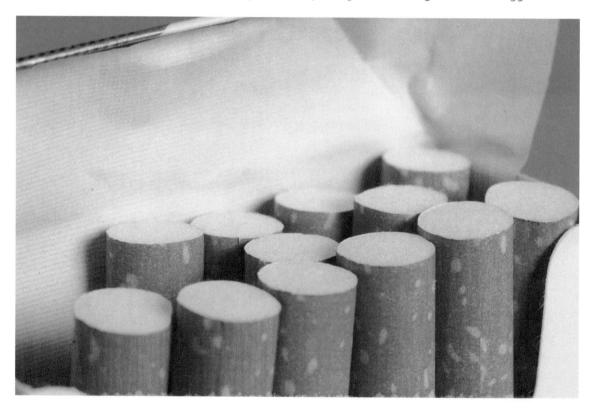

Smoking cigarettes doesn't just affect your sperm, it can also have a big impact on your ability to have sex at all.

In a report by the British Medical Association in 2004, it was revealed that around 120,000 men in their thirties and forties in the UK are impotent as a direct result of smoking.

It's thought that smoking accelerates the process of furring up of the arteries (atherosclerosis), which cuts down the blood flow into the penis needed both to trigger and maintain an erection.

The nicotine in cigarettes also has the effect of causing constriction (tightening) of the walls of these blood vessels, which further reduces this all-important blood flow.

Alcohol

How much booze you drink can have an impact on a number of areas of health, so it won't come as much of a shock to find out that it can also have an impact on how fertile you are. Like smoking, alcohol affects both the quality and quantity of sperm, and as sperm take 72 hours to develop, it can take a while for this damage to be reversed. Fortunately, most of this damage is sustained by men who regularly have a high alcohol intake, so the good news is that the majority of men can avoid this effect simply by taking it easy on the beers.

But alcohol is also renowned for causing impotence (aka 'brewer's droop'), so be aware that binge drinking can affect men's fertility in the short term. Drinking one drink too many may make them feel a bit frisky and decrease their sexual inhibitions, but men won't have much to show for their excitement once they're between the sheets. This means they're probably unlikely to get their leg over, let alone get a leg up in the baby-making stakes.

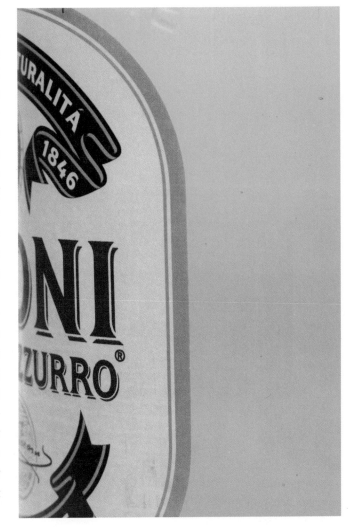

Age

We all know that Charlie Chaplin kept knocking out little ones until he was into his seventies, and there's often a reassuring story in the papers about older celebrities becoming fathers in their sixties (including Sir Paul McCartney, Des O'Connor and Rod Stewart). However, research published in 2006 has shown that it's best not to leave trying for a baby until you're entitled to a bus pass.

Scientists in France looked at almost 2,000 couples who were undergoing fertility treatment and found that 70 per cent of the men who were over the age of just 40 were likely to have problems conceiving. The main culprit for this was again thought to be poor quality sperm, but in men in general another factor seemed to be a declining frequency of sex as they get older.

Temperature

While most men will want a reputation of being hot in the bedroom, there is some evidence to suggest that being hot below the belt is not something to boast about if you want to have a baby.

Testicles hang outside the body for a reason (and it's obviously not an aesthetic one). It is because sperm develop best when they are kept two or three degrees below body temperature. Theoretically then, anything that increases testicular temperature will put a spanner in the works of sperm production, and there is some evidence that increases in testicular temperature of just 1°C can cut down the number of sperm by up to 40 per cent. It's also known that men's sperm counts are lower during the hotter weather of the summer months.

So there's no end of advice around that encourages men to avoid anything that could potentially overheat their goolies: tight underpants, hot baths, laptops and maybe even re-runs of *Charlie's Angels*.

But whether any of this has a direct effect on the chances of conception is the subject of a fair amount of scientific debate – there are obviously tight-pant-wearing laptop users who do have children. So many experts believe that while temperature alone may not dramatically affect a man's fertility, it may prove significant when combined with the other risk factors we've talked about. In which case, wearing boxer shorts and not taking hot baths may be enough to tip the balance in a man's favour and prove to be the difference between becoming a father or not.

Sexually transmitted infections

Sexually transmitted infections such as gonorrhoea and chlamydia have the potential to damage the epididymis and therefore act as a physical blockage to sperm ejaculation. It's therefore always advisable to use a condom when having sex for sex's sake, as it could affect your future chances of having a baby when you do actually want to conceive. If you develop soreness or a discharge from the penis, or pain and irritation when having a pee, see a doctor immediately, as these can be signs that you've picked up an infection.

Diet

We are, apparently, what we eat and if you have a diet lacking in goodness then your body will lack it too, causing all sorts of problems in virtually every system in the body. And that includes the reproductive system.

Fruits containing vitamins C and E, selenium and zinc are thought to be beneficial for fertility. Whether true or not, including fruit and veg in your diet can only do you good.

Some constituents of fruit and veg (particularly vitamins C and E, selenium and zinc) have been mooted as being beneficial to fertility, as they aid sperm production and help repair sperm that have been damaged by our bad habits (such as smoking and drinking). In fact, in 2006, Australian scientists claimed

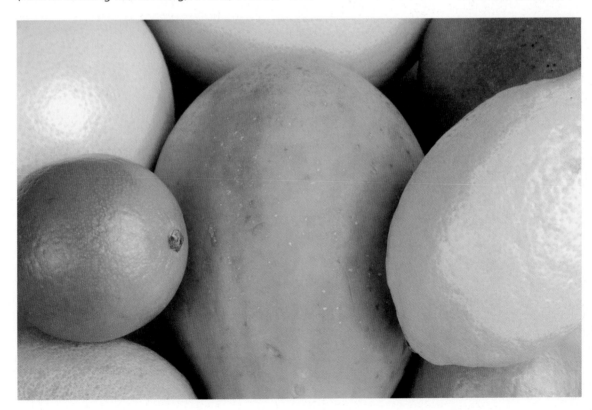

that they had developed a male fertility pill which was made of these and other ingredients which could double the pregnancy rates of infertile couples.

Sounds great, but unfortunately this was a small-scale study of only 60 couples (the bigger the study the better as it helps to rule out chance findings), and it wasn't a randomized controlled trial either. (These are the gold-standard type of clinical trials because they compare whether the treatment is any more

One theory has it that comparing the lengths of a man's ring and index fingers on his right hand will indicate his level of fertility.

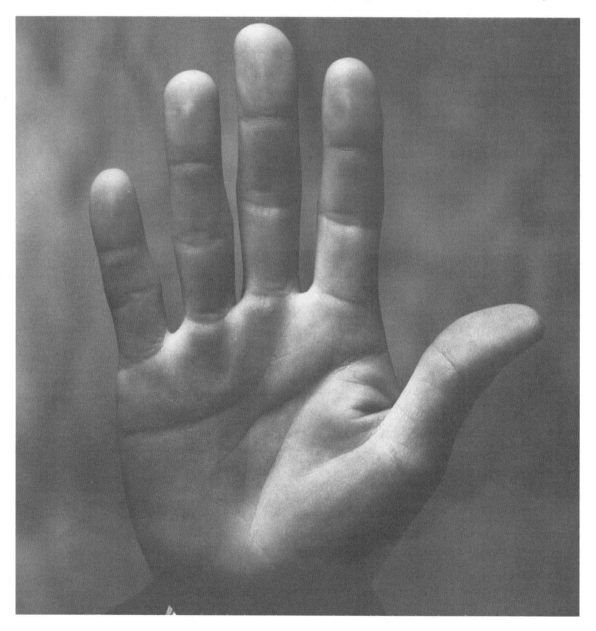

effective than a placebo sugar pill.) So, sadly, at the moment these results are a little unconvincing.

There's also not a lot of hard evidence to support dosing up on these vitamin and mineral pills individually either. So despite the fact that you will be bombarded by pop-ups advertising these supplements every time you visit a fertility website, you're better off saving your money and just eating your greens. It's a more natural way to absorb vitamins and minerals and it keeps you regular too!

Sexual lubricants

A few studies have looked at the effect of commonly used vaginal lubricants on the mobility of sperm, and the results have shown that they are generally best avoided. Tests have been carried out on lubricant jelly, saliva, baby oil and olive oil and all but baby oil have been found to reduce the amount of sperm movement significantly.

Therefore it is advisable to steer clear of using vaginal lubricants when trying for a baby if possible, and perhaps to avoid oral sex as well, given the negative impact that saliva seems to have on sperm.

Digit length

This is probably the most fascinating of all the factors that it has ever been claimed are critical to a man's sperm production – and if it does turn out to be important, there's not a lot you can do about this one!

It has been suggested by scientists (most notably the British evolutionary psychologist Dr John Manning) that the ratio of the length of the index and ring fingers (first and third fingers) on a man's right hand is affected by the amount of testosterone that he was exposed to as a baby in the womb.

In general, men have a longer third finger than index finger and in women the lengths are either equal or the other way around (with the index finger being the longest). However, in a study published in 1998, Manning and his colleagues found that men whose first finger on their right hand was longer than their third had lower testosterone levels and sperm counts than those whose ratio was more common.

More research is obviously needed to see whether this has any bearing on fertility in real life, but it's obviously food for thought. However, I must say I'm a little bit sceptical about this theory, since my right third finger is longer than my first, and yet I have three children.

Female fertility

A woman's fertility, as you'd no doubt expect, is a little more complex than that of a man. Here there are two main areas involved, either of which can cause difficulties. Firstly, there's the ovulation process: if there's no egg, then there's nothing for a sperm to fertilize. Secondly, there's the reproductive tract (vagina, uterus, fallopian tubes) which can be obstructed at any point along its route and so, therefore, can literally stop the sperm in their tracks.

Lifestyle factors

Just as with a man's fertility, there are a number of lifestyle issues which can affect a woman's ability to conceive. Some of these will affect the production of eggs during the monthly menstrual cycle, while others can cause damage to the reproductive tract, thereby preventing any incoming sperm from reaching their target.

Weight

As with men, carrying too much or not enough weight can be a problem. Experts advise that an optimum BMI for conception is somewhere between 19 and 28. Drop above or below these figures and you could encounter a few problems:

- **Low bodyweight** – Our bodies are equipped with some wonderful survival mechanisms to protect us against extreme conditions, but as these are out of our direct control they can sometimes become a disadvantage.

  Take weight loss, for example. If you lose too much weight your body thinks you're experiencing famine conditions and will stop your reproductive cycle, because there's no point producing offspring who are certain to die of starvation. In developed countries this type of weight loss is more likely to be self-inflicted – by extreme dieting or obsessional exercise for instance – and there are lots of cases of female athletes whose periods have stopped, not because of environmental dangers, but because their bodies couldn't cope with making a baby.

- **Obesity** – Being significantly overweight is as bad news as being underweight when it comes to trying for a baby. Fat cells in the body make hormones which can, when produced in sufficient quantities (as they will be if there's lots of fat around), interfere with normal cycles and so prevent ovulation from occurring.

  Obesity is also a significant risk factor for first trimester miscarriage.

A crucial fertility issue for women is weight, but diets should be followed carefully, as losing too much weight can have an adverse effect.

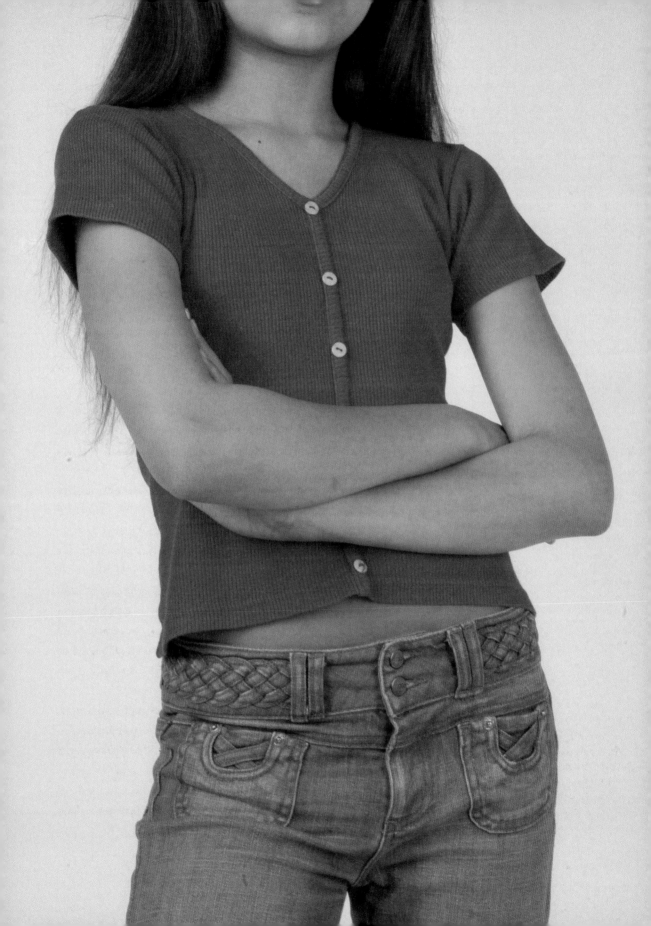

Smoking

Ta dah! Here's a shock, smoking is bad news for female fertility too. When Dutch scientists looked at 8,000 women who were undergoing fertility treatment, they found that women who smoked were 28 per cent less likely to have a baby than those who didn't. They also concluded that by smoking a woman is kissing goodbye to ten years of her reproductive life – so a 30-year-old smoker reduces her chances of being a mum to those of a 40-year-old (see age-related statistics below). If you're a smoker who's already nearly 40, then that's really not good news, because your chances of becoming pregnant will dip even further still.

Other research makes even gloomier reading. Doctors who have studied couples trying for a baby naturally (so not those under fertility specialists like the women in the Dutch research) have found that 42 per cent of smokers take more than a year to become pregnant.

Alcohol

As with men, alcohol can make women less fertile. It's thought that this is because it increases the level of oestrogen in women's bodies, therefore switching off production of the hormone FSH in the brain, which in turn lowers the chances of ovulation each month (see page 14).

Alcohol also affects progesterone levels, which may prevent the successful implantation of fertilized eggs in the womb, resulting in a higher chance of miscarriage.

Age

From the moment she starts her periods a woman's biological clock is ticking, and the older she gets, the louder the ticking becomes. So, whereas women aged between 19 and 26 have around a 50 per cent chance of pregnancy in any one menstrual cycle, for women aged 27 to 34 that chance has dropped to 40 per cent. For those in the next age bracket – from 35 to 39 – it has plummeted a further 10 per cent to less than 30 per cent per menstrual cycle.

So as far as the amount of time it generally takes to conceive is concerned, it's thought that it can be around three to four months for an average, healthy, 25-year-old woman, then twice this for someone who is 35, while by the age of 39 this has rocketed to 15 months.

There's a heap of reasons why this might happen, including less regular ovulation and a greater risk of damaged chromosomes inside her eggs (which leads to a failure of implantation and a higher chance of miscarriage). It's also thought that a woman's sex drive decreases as she becomes older, which will also have a detrimental effect on her chances of conceiving.

Sexually transmitted infections

Unlike the reasons above, sexually transmitted infections don't upset the menstrual cycle; however, they do pose a risk to a woman's fertility by potentially blocking her tubes. The main culprit here is chlamydia, which has become a frighteningly common infection in younger women, with a doubling in cases in the five years

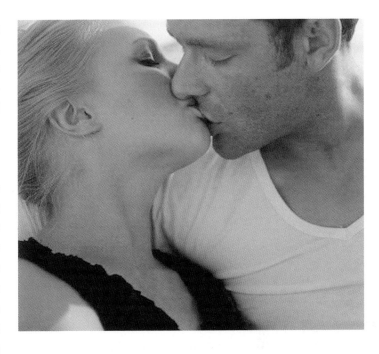

between 1997 and 2002. As a result, it's now thought that one in ten sexually active women under the age of 25 are infected.

Chlamydia is having a field day amongst young, sexually active women these days. It can be treated if spotted early, but if it is left it can have a devastating effect on fertility.

This is obviously great news if you are a chlamydia bug, because as part of a very successful species you have the best possible chance of a long and happy life. It's not such good news for our species, though, with some experts claiming that up to one-third of all women who need fertility treatment require it because of damage caused by this bacterium.

Chlamydia is not always that easy to diagnose either, because three-quarters of women who have this infection (it's caught by having unprotected sex with an infected man) don't have any symptoms. Those women who do show signs may notice that they have an abnormal vaginal discharge, discomfort when peeing, pelvic pain and sometimes pain during sex. So this infection is diagnosed either by taking swabs from the cervix (neck of the womb) or from testing a sample of urine. The good news is that it can be treated quite straightforwardly with a course of antibiotics. However, those people whose infection lies undetected – and therefore untreated – are at risk of scarring of their fallopian tubes, which not only reduces fertility but carries a high risk of an ectopic pregnancy if conception does occur.

The bottom line here is: always make him use a condom and see a doctor if you have the first inkling of any of the symptoms of an STI.

Diet

As with men, the evidence for fertile properties of certain foods is weak, and the advice is to eat a well-balanced diet with at least five portions of fruit and vegetables to keep yourself healthy and at the ideal weight.

Contraception

It doesn't take a genius to work out that in order to conceive you have to stop using contraception; but some contraceptives that you've used in the past can take a while to get out of your system and so they could slow you down in your rush to have a baby.

This is particularly true for contraceptive injections and after long-term use of the combined contraceptive pill. The mini pill and the coil have little effect, as, obviously, do condoms. But the impact of contraception doesn't last long and most likely only means that it takes a couple of cycles for you to start ovulating again and get your body ready to conceive. In a reassuring study of 750 women in Germany, published in 2006, it was found that over the course of a year, the conception rate for women who had used these birth control methods was identical to that of women who'd never used contraception (around 85 per cent)

Until you dispense with contraception in order to have a baby, condoms will protect you and your fertility from damaging sexual diseases.

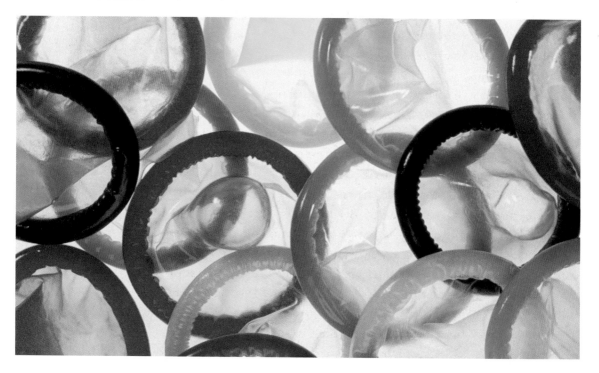

Getting down to business

So you've made the decision to have a baby and you're primed for conception now that you've heeded all the advice above. Your body is a lean, mean breeding machine, and all you have to do is to have sex and the rest of the process should take care of itself.

Well, sort of. You can, of course, just randomly start having it off like rabbits, cross your fingers and hope that that works – and in a high percentage of cases it will. There's absolutely nothing wrong with that approach, and by being so relaxed about it all it's bound to make the process less stressful and a lot more fun.

However, there are a number of things you can do if you prefer to hedge your bets and save your energies for times when you're most likely to strike it lucky. In fact, there's no shortage of advice out there about how to maximize your chances of success: by planning how often you should do it, when in your cycle you should be trying your hardest, and the best positions to contort yourselves into while you're on the job. Unfortunately some of this advice, which is largely based on old wives' tales, is at best misguided and at worst complete pants.

So here's a round-up of the best evidence available with the scientific wheat sorted from the unscientific, mumbo-jumbo-laden chaff. Old wives look away.

Fertile window

As a woman, the first thing you need to do is to get to know your fertile window. This is not to be mistaken for the Fertile Crescent in the Middle East, which you'll have learned about in your school geography lessons (as this will obviously be of no help at all), but is instead the period during the menstrual cycle when your chance of conceiving is at its highest. In other words, the time when it's most likely that your partner's sperm will find an egg ready and waiting for them.

In the past it was believed that this window of opportunity only occurred on the day of ovulation itself, so many couples wasted their efforts going at it hell for leather on that day alone only to be disappointed by the appearance of a normal period a couple of weeks later.

The reason that many couples do not succeed in getting pregnant on this one day is because each egg is only viable for 24 hours. So, by adopting this course of action you are placing a severe restriction on your chances, as you might find yourself only able to have sex at a time when

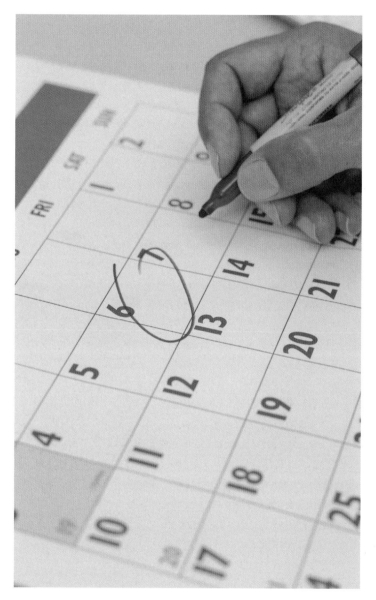

If you have a regular menstrual cycle, or know your cycle well, you can work out the best time for those romantic nights in.

the egg is past its best. Sperm, on the other hand, can last for up to six days (although as we've seen they'll suffer heavy losses during that time), so given their longevity the evidence suggests that the fertile window actually begins about five days before ovulation and ends on the day of ovulation itself.

For maximum success, however, you should particularly be aiming to have sex around two days before ovulation when the sperm are still fresh and not too battle-weary.

Pinpointing ovulation

Of course, in order to be able to calculate your fertile window you need to be able to predict when it is that you'll ovulate. In a textbook 28-day menstrual cycle, ovulation occurs 14 days before the first day of your next period – and if you're a textbook type of girl who's as regular as clockwork, it's not too tricky to do the maths.

Women's cycles do, of course, vary, with some being shorter than 28 days and others lasting for up to 35 days. But in either case, as long as you're regular, the calculation is the same – if you have a 35-day cycle, for instance, count 14 days backwards from your period and you can put ovulation at around day 21, one whole week later than for a woman with a 28-day cycle.

The difficulty comes when your cycles are completely random and last, say, 24 days one month but 32 the next. In this situation, how do you know when your egg is ready? You could just take an average and work out ovulation that way, but that will be a bit hit and miss. So instead you might try one of the commonly used methods for predicting ovulation, which are based on observing the changes that happen in your body as that all-important time approaches.

Body temperature

This is a haphazard and unreliable method that verges on old wives' territory. The theory goes that just prior to ovulation your body temperature dips, only to rise again sharply 24 hours after ovulation. So by charting your temperature for a number of months you should, theoretically, be able to pinpoint when you ovulate.

However, in many women this temperature rise occurs several days after ovulation, which makes it virtually impossible to determine the exact date; so it's not a method worth wasting time on.

Cervical mucus

This method was developed by two Australian doctors in the 1970s and relies on the fact that about five or six days before ovulation the mucus in the cervix, and hence vaginal discharge, becomes clear and stretchy (a bit like egg white). This mucus helps sperm travel through the female reproductive system, so starting to have sex once this appears should allow you to identify your fertile window and thereby improve your chances of conception.

A number of studies have looked at the effectiveness of this method and the general belief is that if you can learn to be confident in identifying this type of cervical mucus, then you could actually double your chances of conceiving during that cycle.

Ovulation kits

There are a number of kits on the market that allow you to test samples of your urine for levels of luteinizing hormone (LH). This hormone has a surge in its level a day or two before ovulation, so this allows the manufacturers of these kits to claim that their products can help couples identify the best days on which to conceive a baby.

Unfortunately, some studies have shown that this is not 100 per cent reliable for women whose cycles are less than 21 days or greater than 42 days, and that the two days identified may not be the days of highest probability of conception during the fertile window. So more research is obviously needed to assess their true effectiveness. However, for many women such ovulation kits can serve as a useful guide.

Frequency of sex

You now know when to have sex, but how often should you be doing it?

This question is more pertinent for the male half of the fertility equation than the female, as it's crucial that each time a man has sex he has enough sperm to ejaculate if he is going to have a fair chance of making his efforts count.

There's a popular myth that says that if men abstain from sex and store up their sperm then they will become more potent at key times. In fact the opposite is true: if you keep sperm hanging around they will eventually begin to crowd each other out and get fed up with sharing resources. It's a bit like when people have to wait in airport departure lounges during air traffic control strikes: they start out fresh but eventually run out of space and provisions and end up exhausted. So after 14 days of abstention there are likely to be less than 7 per cent motile sperm left.

On the other hand, you don't want to go mad and have sex every five minutes either, because if you do you'll quickly use up all of your sperm. (You certainly don't want to waste them on DIY sex while you're trying for a baby, because if you masturbate twice in a day before having sex with your partner you'll use up around 75 per cent of your available sperm.) So having sex every other day during the fertile period is probably about right for making sure your sperm are in reasonable nick and up to the job of reaching and fertilizing that egg.

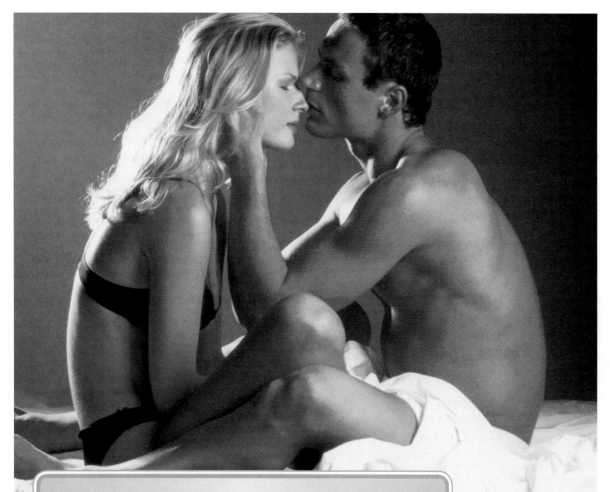

CONCEPTUAL KAMA SUTRA

The ancient Indian text, the *Kama Sutra*, is a guidebook for sexual behaviour, and in its most famous chapters it contains details of 64 different sexual positions that can be adopted without the need for extraneous paraphernalia. And to be honest there's absolutely no reason why you shouldn't try to work your way through the lot of them when you're trying for a baby.

Of course, we're not all equally flexible and you may find some of the positions impossible to achieve without the aid of a safety net and some surgical appliances. But remember that sex for reproduction shouldn't be a chore – so try to have some fun along the way.

Conceiving can take time, so don't let sex become a chore – keep it fun and interesting.

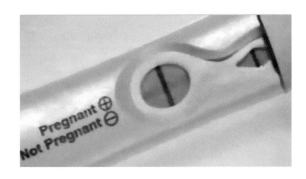

The wait for that little blue line takes only a few minutes, but it can feel like an eternity.

The whole process of trying for a baby can be quicker than a blink of the eye, or it can be long and stressful. Remember to keep calm and relaxed about it and don't let every period that arrives get you down. Pep up your sex life and try not to let it become simply a means to an end; experiment with different positions and make it fun.

As far as chances of success are concerned, positions which allow deep penetration to occur are more likely to lead to conception because sperm is deposited close to the cervix, whereas positions where the woman is on top are more likely to increase flowback and loss of sperm. Despite that, there's not a lot of evidence to promote the practice of putting a pillow under the woman's bum or getting her to do handstands after sex to keep the sperm in.

Even if you do know all the tricks of the trade and follow all these theories to the letter, it is still not unusual for couples to take two years to conceive. If after that time (or after one year for those women over 35) nothing seems to be working, then it might be time to go and see your doctor who can refer you to a specialist for further investigation.

Low sperm count

Although there are a number of tips couples can follow to maximize their chances of breeding success, there are some problems that can seem insurmountable and extremely depressing. For men this can be the realization that they have insufficient healthy sperm to fertilize their partner's eggs.

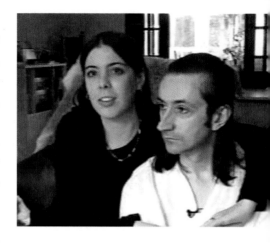

In *Make Me a Baby,* all the men collected a sperm sample for analysis which was used to help them assess their chances of becoming fathers. For some this was reassuring but for others, like Paul, the result came as quite a shock.

Paul's sperm count put him right down at the low end of the range and went some way to explaining why, despite the fact that he and his wife Juliet were both very healthy, non-smokers of normal weight, they'd been trying for a baby for months with no success.

Armed with this result, Paul booked an appointment with a local fertility clinic for further tests to see if they too would show this problem and confirm the findings of his first test. They did.

Through discussions with the medical team it transpired that, as a boy, Paul had had a condition called torsion of the testes (where one of the testicles twists inside the scrotum, cutting off its blood supply and potentially affecting future sperm production), which he had never before been told about.

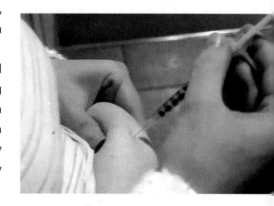

So Paul and Juliet were advised that their best chance of conceiving was by a form of invitro fertilisation (IVF) called Intracytoplasmic sperm injection (ICSI), which is particularly helpful when infertility is caused by sperm problems.

This procedure begins by stimulating the ovaries of the woman using a hormone injection annd then collecting the eggs which are produced. These injections go just under the skin and are usually administered by the woman herself.

After around two weeks of these jabs the number of eggs produced is assessed in the clinic using a vaginal ultrasound scan. Once the doctors are happy that the process has been a success, the eggs are collected using a probe which passes through the vagina, guided along by ultrasound equipment.

The male partner provides a sperm sample on the same day that the eggs are collected. This is usually done by masturbation, although if a man has no viable sperm at all, sperm can be collected from the testes themselves.

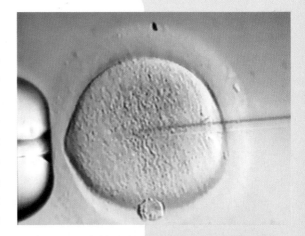

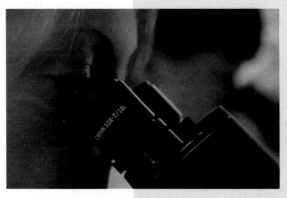

Next the sperm are injected directly into the eggs (one sperm per egg) and are left in an incubator overnight to see if any of the eggs become fertilized. Three or four which successfully fertilize will then be left for a further day to develop before being placed into the woman's womb.

Couples undergoing all forms of IVF, including ICSI, have a one in five chance of conceiving at the first attempt, with success being greater for those who are under 35. In many parts of the country this treatment is available on the NHS, but thanks to the infamous postcode lottery of fertility services (it's available from some NHS trusts and not others), many couples find it extremely difficult to benefit from it and will be forced to undergo costly private treatment.

In their first ICSI treatment Juliet and Paul had 14 eggs collected, but only two embryos made it through the night. Sadly these two didn't implant in Juliet's womb. Despite this disappointment, Paul and Juliet have decided to keep trying with the treatment and plan to repeat it in the near future in the hope of conceiving.

In order to conceive a much-wanted baby, Paul and Juliet have gone through the process of invitro fertilization. This involved Juliet administering regular injections into her tummy to stimulate her ovaries. Her eggs were then injected with Paul's sperm under a microscope before the successfully fertilized embryos were returned to Juliet's womb.

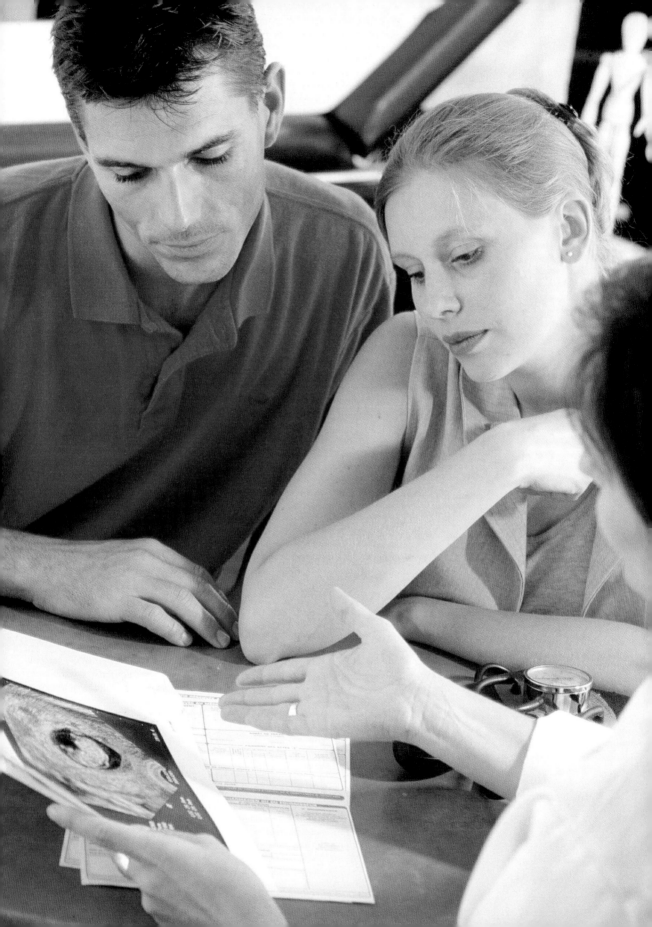

chapter 2

Early pregnancy

Most women can sail through pregnancy quite comfortably without needing to come within one hundred miles of any trained specialists. After all, our species did manage to breed successfully for many millennia without the assistance of midwives, doctors and ultrasound scanners.

That said, however, pregnancy can provide you with an assortment of troublesome symptoms, and there's a small possibility of some potentially serious (but thankfully uncommon) complications that can threaten the health of you and your baby. For this reason, antenatal care has been devised as a way of keeping an eye on a woman throughout her pregnancy; to ensure that it runs as smoothly as possible and also to help her prepare for the impending sleepless world of parenthood.

Antenatal care

Most antenatal care is provided within the community, rather than in hospital units. In the majority of cases a midwife will be the key health professional involved, but your care will probably be shared with your GP. However, a referral to an obstetrician will be arranged should any problems arise during the course of your pregnancy which require more specialist monitoring. This care will take the form of a series of visits to your healthcare specialists.

First-time mums who experience a trouble-free pregnancy, however, can expect to have to pitch up for a clinic visit around ten times before they give birth, whereas those who've been there, done that (and have a weaker pelvic floor to prove it!) should expect around seven appointments – providing their previous pregnancy or pregnancies were uncomplicated.

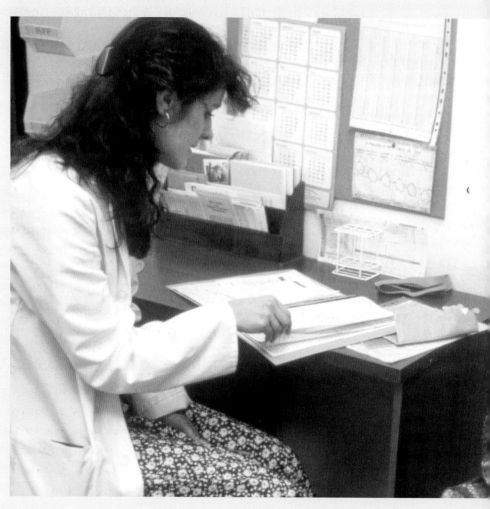

What to expect at the first appointment

The first doctor's appointment that you attend is likely to be the one in which you announce that you've had a positive pregnancy test and ask the doctor what on earth happens next. Even if the pregnancy is planned, the realization that the time you have spent trying has finally paid off can be quite scary; and if it's an unplanned baby your anxiety can verge on blind panic.

So on this first visit your doctor will confirm that you have taken a pregnancy test and will also ask you the date on which your last period began. This information is important because pregnancy is estimated as 40 weeks from the first day of your last period, so by knowing when this was the doctor can work out your expected date of delivery (or EDD). This can give you a guide as to when you might expect to hear the patter of tiny feet.

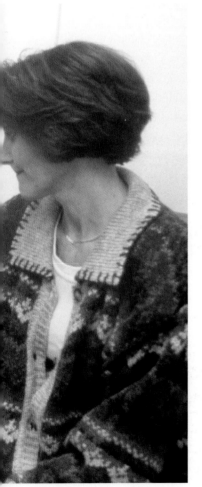

However, if you have an erratic menstrual cycle and you are unsure of when your last period was, the doctor might arrange an early dating ultrasound scan to see where you are in your pregnancy and, therefore, give you a more accurate idea of when your baby might put in an appearance.

In the olden days the doctor would also don a pair of latex gloves and embark upon an internal examination, but this is a rare occurrence now and this first appointment is usually just a cosy and, hopefully, reassuring chat. In this conversation your doctor will probably outline some of the dos and don'ts of early pregnancy (see pages 50 and 51), discuss any early symptoms that you've had – such as sore breasts, tiredness, nausea and the constant urge to head for the loo – and will check you're taking the folic acid tablets recommended for expectant mothers until the 12th week of pregnancy.

Much of what happens at this first appointment will probably be a blur, but you'll hopefully leave the surgery feeling a lot calmer than when you arrived. You will also come away with an appointment date to see the midwife, a prescription for folic acid (if you need one) and a rough plan of how events will unfold over the next nine months of your life.

Your first appointment will involve more paperwork than physical tests, but it's an important start to the pregnancy journey.

Choosing where to have your baby

Most people these days opt to give birth in hospital (only around 12,000 babies are delivered at home per year). This decision is usually made because of the reassurance of being surrounded by trained staff and lots of high-tech wizardry – and also because there's someone else there to clean up the mess afterwards. In many areas the choice of maternity unit is limited to just one hospital, but sometimes there will be alternatives on offer. Which one you pick will depend on a number of factors, including your own past experiences of a particular hospital or those of your friends and family. Your decision may also be dictated by any problems you've had during your pregnancy and whether these demand the expertise of a particular unit.

Proximity to home is an important consideration when choosing where to give birth; the last thing you need when you're in the painful throes of labour is a long journey with the inherent risk that you may end up giving birth in a lay-by.

Your midwife can talk you through the pros and cons of what's available and you may also be able to visit your local units to have a poke around before you make up your mind. Independent advice is also available from an organization called Dr Foster, which has facts and figures relating to all maternity units in the country (see the website www.drfoster.co.uk).

However, home births are an attractive option for those with an uncomplicated pregnancy or for those who are not having their first baby and so are more confident about the whole birth experience. Home births have the advantage of allowing you to deliver your baby in comfortable, less clinical surroundings where the whole family can be involved, if you wish. There are no bags to pack, no frantic dash to hospital and, if it floats your boat, the unique possibility of delivering in a nest of cushions surrounded by soothing sounds while calming scents waft your baby into the outside world.

What you can't have, of course, is an epidural, and other than the gas and air that your midwife will provide, pain relief will rely heavily on the atmosphere of your surroundings and a heavy dose of mind over matter.

That said, many women find it a more 'enjoyable' experience because of, rather than in spite of, this reduced medical involvement. (A fact endorsed by my own mother who popped me out *au naturel* on to the eiderdown in my Nan's back bedroom.)

Before you make great plans for a home birth, though, be warned that there are certain situations in which doctors will be keen to veto your plans in order to safeguard your health, that of your baby, or both:

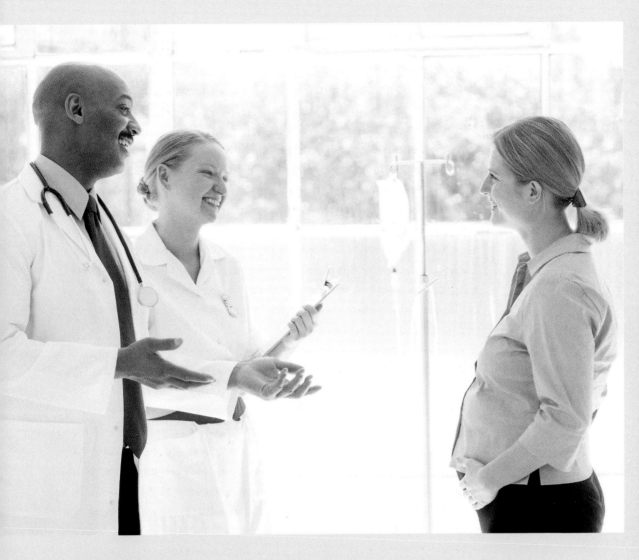

- Breech presentation.
- Multiple pregnancy (having twins or triplets, etc.).
- Antepartum haemorrhage.
- Pre-eclampsia.
- Intrauterine growth retardation (babies may be small because the placenta isn't working well and will need careful monitoring).
- Previous Caesarean section.
- Gestational diabetes.
- You have a heart condition.
- There have been any antenatal complications.

A hospital birth is recommended for any woman experiencing a problematic pregnancy, but it will also give you the reassurance of having experienced medical care and facilities close to hand should you need it.

Booking appointment

This is the first time that you'll get to meet your midwife, who should (hopefully) stay with you throughout the pregnancy, but won't necessarily deliver your baby – unless you have a home birth. During this appointment, which is likely to be the longest that you will have to endure, she will want full details of your medical and family history and information about any previous pregnancies.

All of this information will be recorded in a book which you will be given to keep with you throughout your pregnancy and which will be updated along the way with test and scan results, as well as with medical notes from clinic or hospital visits. It is a good idea always to have this book handy and you should even take it away on holiday with you – just in case you need medical assistance in an emergency.

To make sure your notes are as comprehensive as possible, your midwife will pry into almost every aspect of your lifestyle. She will check up on your smoking, drinking, illicit drug use and dietary habits, find out what sort of

PREGNANCY DOS AND DON'TS

DO

⬧ Take folic acid tablets: they help to protect against health problems for the baby such as spina bifida. If you are planning a pregnancy, take these tablets as soon as you start trying for a baby. They're available over the counter at all pharmacies and the recommended dose is 400 micrograms per day.

⬧ Carry on exercising – moderate exercise is quite safe but contact sports, scuba diving and sports that risk abdominal trauma should be avoided.

⬧ Eat a healthy, well-balanced diet.

⬧ Carry on working – unless your doctor has advised you not to.

⬧ Visit the dentist for a free check up.

⬧ Have sex – if you feel like it! You might have to adjust positions as your body shape changes, but sex won't do your baby any harm.

⬧ Have holidays, but do also remember that air travel carries an increased risk of deep vein thrombosis and many airlines will not allow women to fly if they are 36 weeks pregnant or over. The safest time for air travel is believed to be between 18 and 24 weeks.

⬧ Put a car seatbelt above and below your bump – not on top of it.

DON'T

- Take vitamin A supplements or eat liver (which contains high levels of this vitamin) as it can affect your baby's development and can cause a higher risk of your baby having defects of its head, brain and heart.

- Drink unpasteurized milk, eat blue or soft cheeses (e.g., brie and camembert), pâté or undercooked meals which could carry listeria, an infection which can lead to miscarriage or stillbirth.

- Eat more than two tuna steaks or four medium-sized tins of tuna per week, because although the levels of mercury in this food have no effect on adults they can affect a baby's developing nervous system.

- Eat raw or partially cooked eggs (including real mayonnaise), or raw or partially cooked meat as these can carry salmonella, which is an infection that can be passed on to the foetus.

- Take medicines or alternative remedies (other than paracetamol) that have not been prescribed by your doctor or homeopath.

- Drink more than one unit of alcohol per day (one unit is a small glass of wine, half a pint of standard strength beer or cider, or a standard measure of spirits). Alcohol can cross into the placenta and if consumed regularly in large doses can lead to a baby having growth and mental retardation, behavioural problems and facial and heart defects.

- Smoke, as it can have a severe impact on a newborn's health. Smoking increases the risk of premature delivery and of having a

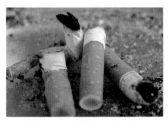

low birthweight baby. Both of these effects put a baby at extra risk of anatomical abnormalities, asphyxia at birth, severe low blood sugar and a predisposition to developing diabetes.

- Use street drugs: these can cause premature birth, miscarriage and serious defects in your baby. Babies of drug users can also be born with their own addictions to a drug.

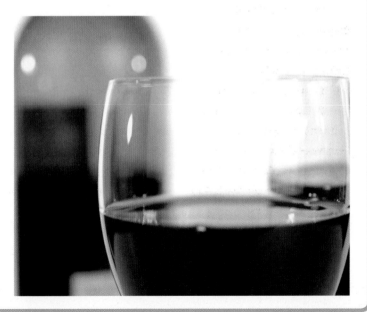

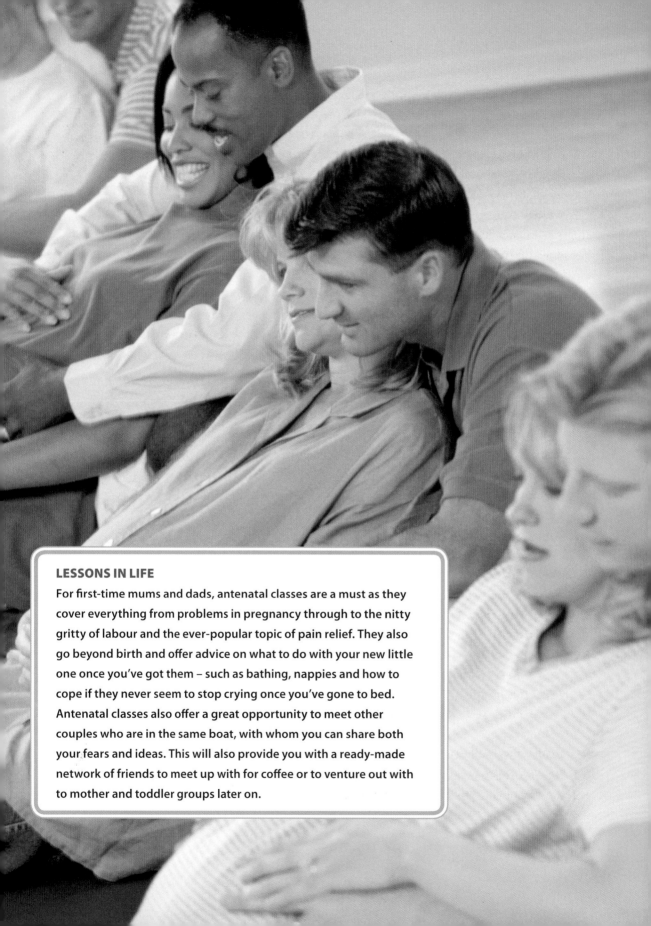

LESSONS IN LIFE

For first-time mums and dads, antenatal classes are a must as they cover everything from problems in pregnancy through to the nitty gritty of labour and the ever-popular topic of pain relief. They also go beyond birth and offer advice on what to do with your new little one once you've got them – such as bathing, nappies and how to cope if they never seem to stop crying once you've gone to bed. Antenatal classes also offer a great opportunity to meet other couples who are in the same boat, with whom you can share both your fears and ideas. This will also provide you with a ready-made network of friends to meet up with for coffee or to venture out with to mother and toddler groups later on.

exercise (if any) you do, what your occupation is, whether you've had any sexually transmitted infections, any terminations (abortions) or miscarriages. She will need to know if you have any chronic illnesses – such as high blood pressure, asthma, diabetes or epilepsy – and if there's anything that you are allergic to. Your midwife will also want a full list of prescription medications that you might take or potions that you regularly pick up from the herbalist. And, of course, she'll also ask you whether there are any twins or genetic conditions in your family. In fact, short of taking your inside leg measurement and finding out where you had your first kiss, she should know everything about you by the time she's finished.

Once all of that is out of the way, your midwife will probably give you a selection of booklets and leaflets with useful information about pregnancy and birth. She will also discuss a plan for your remaining antenatal care and tell you about the maternity benefits that are available to you, depending on your personal and financial situation.

At this appointment your midwife should also let you know about the antenatal classes running in your area – either provided privately or through the NHS. Many of these classes will also offer trips to the local maternity unit so that you can familiarize yourself with these rather clinical surroundings before the big day itself. If, however, you are planning to have your baby in your own front room, your midwife will take you through all the ins and outs of having a home birth, too.

Finally, the midwife will whip out her blood-taking needle and will extract enough blood to fill a variety of pots to run some basic checks. These tests will include:

- A full blood count to look for anaemia.
- A check of your blood group and rhesus status.
- A screen for infections such as rubella (German measles), syphilis, hepatitis and HIV.
- Electrophoresis, which is a test offered to mothers of Asian, Afro-Caribbean or Mediterranean origin who are more at risk of being carriers of genetic conditions such as thalassaemia and sickle-cell anaemia.

(A word of reassurance to new mothers-to-be who have a pathological fear of needles: blood will be taken at several antenatal appointments, and so by the end of your pregnancy you will probably have overcome your phobia and be positively blasé about the whole process!)

Antenatal classes are invaluable opportunities for you and your partner to learn about pregnancy, birth and the early days of caring for your baby.

BLOOD GROUPS

Blood groups are determined by the types of protein molecules (called antigens) we have on the walls of our red blood cells. These form specific patterns and allow us to classify the main blood types into A, B and O groups.

People with blood group A have the A-pattern proteins on all of their red cells; those in group B have the B pattern; those in group AB have (surprise, surprise) both A and B; and finally, people with blood group O have neither A nor B. Blood groups cause few problems in pregnancy, but it's important information to have in case you need a blood transfusion – as some can clash with each other and cause potentially life-threatening complications if they are inadvertently mixed.

The other main blood group classification is called the rhesus system. Again, this is down to patterns of proteins on red blood cells, but this time there are at least 40 varieties. The most important of these is the D group: if you have this pattern then you are rhesus positive; if not, you're rhesus negative.

Problems can arise in pregnancy when a rhesus negative mother is expecting a rhesus positive baby and becomes sensitized to its blood cells. This usually happens if there's bleeding in the womb, such as during a threatened miscarriage or during a technical procedure like an amniocentesis. In this situation the mother can potentially make antibodies which can attack the baby's blood cells and burst them, causing a condition known as haemolytic anaemia.

This is bad news for the foetus, which runs the risk of developing an extensive list of particularly nasty complications, such as hypoxia (low oxygen), liver and heart dysfunction, growth restriction, limited movement and generalized fluid overload in all its tissues so that it's skin, lungs and belly become literally waterlogged. Babies who develop haemolytic anaemia need to be treated in specialized hospital units, where they may need a blood transfusion while still inside the womb.

The good news is that by checking on all women's blood groups, this can usually be avoided by giving at-risk mums a dose of what's called anti-D. This stops the sensitization and the subsequent production of antibodies and nips the whole process in the bud.

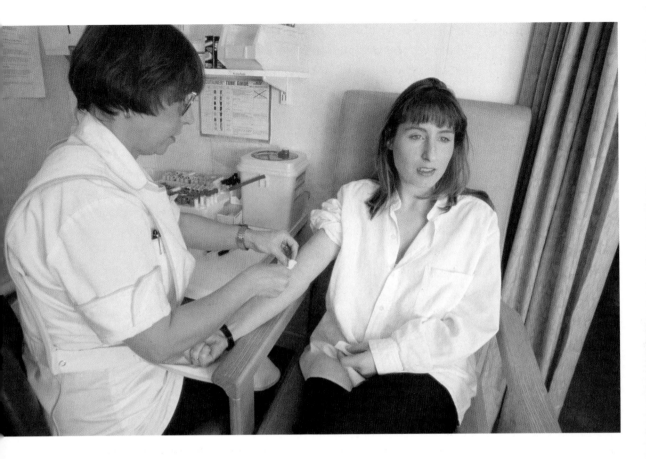

Further appointments

After these initial appointments you will continue to have regular catch-ups with your midwife and your GP until you go into labour. These appointments are arranged so they can keep an eye on the mother and also the development of the baby. In order to make sure that everything is progressing normally, you will experience a series of checks at various times. These include:

Blood pressure: It's important to measure this from the start of your pregnancy because rises in blood pressure over the nine months can sometimes be a sign of pre-eclampsia (see page 113).

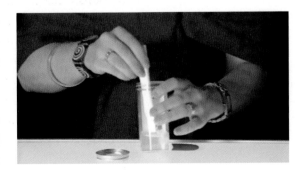

Urine sample: A pot of this stuff will be your constant companion to antenatal appointments, and at each one the midwife or doctor will test it with a

The distance between the symphysis pubis and the top of your womb should increase by roughly 1cm per week. This measurement allows your doctor to determine how well your baby is growing.

dipstick for traces of blood, protein and glucose. Protein can be an early indicator of pre-eclampsia, and if it is combined with a microscopic trace of blood and you are experiencing pain when you pee, it could be that the mother has a urinary tract infection. These are more common in pregnancy because the growing womb can make the bladder drain more slowly, and if left untreated they can trigger premature labour. The appearance of glucose in urine isn't usually a cause for concern as it is common, especially after meals, because the kidneys become relatively leaky during pregnancy and more gets into your urine than you would normally expect. However, if this persists or if glucose is present in large quantities it can mean that you are developing diabetes, in which case you will be advised to undergo a glucose tolerance test.

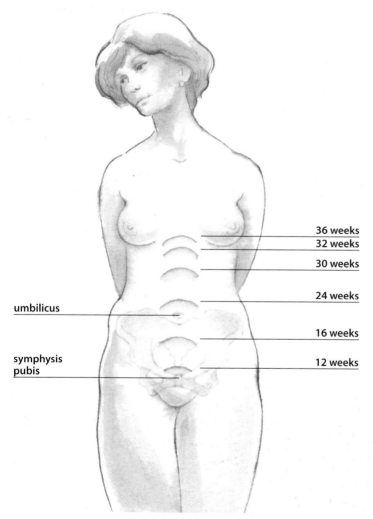

umbilicus

symphysis pubis

36 weeks
32 weeks
30 weeks
24 weeks
16 weeks
12 weeks

Abdominal size: The distance between your symphysis pubis and the top of your womb (see diagram) indicates how your baby is growing. This distance will increase by approximately one centimetre every week until you reach 36 weeks, when the head moves down into the pelvis and prepares to pop out, dropping the height of your bump.

Foetal movements: You will probably begin feeling these at around 20 weeks in a first pregnancy, but often sooner in subsequent ones. (This time was historically known by the rather poetic term 'the quickening'.) It is usual to feel several movements each hour, but if this doesn't happen then you may be asked to keep a kick chart. For this you will start recording movements at 9 a.m. and contact the midwife if you have not felt ten kicks by mid-afternoon. Usually this offers sufficient reassurance that all is well because the perceived lack of movement is often due to the fact that you've been too busy to notice. If, however, less than ten movements are recorded then you might be sent to the hospital for a more detailed assessment, where you will be linked up to a cardiotocograph machine which will monitor the baby's activities. (See page 157.)

Foetal heartbeat: The sound of your baby's heartbeat is one of the most magical sounds that you will ever hear. Doctors used to check this with a pinnard stethoscope (below) which reassured them the baby was behaving itself, but it was completely inaudible to the mother. Nowadays a doctor will check the heart with a sonicaid or doppler device which not only picks up the heartbeat but also broadcasts it to everyone in the room.

In days gone by the pinnard stethoscope only allowed your doctor to hear your baby's heartbeat, but now you can share the experience.

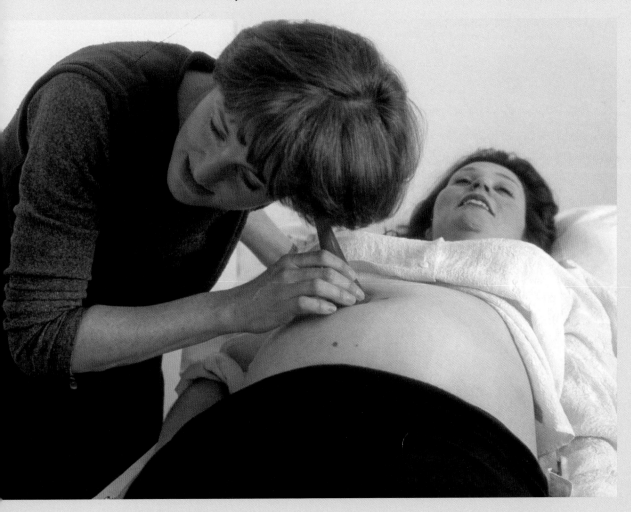

Common complaints in the first trimester

Although pregnancy is not a disease, it is a period of time that can be plagued by irritating or uncomfortable ailments. These are some of the most common ones that you might experience.

Morning sickness

Up to 70 per cent of mothers-to-be are afflicted by morning sickness in early pregnancy. The nausea begins at around six weeks and generally wears off between 12 and 16 weeks, although for some poor souls it can hang around right up until delivery.

Morning sickness can be a bit of an understatement as for many women it can strike at any time or even last the whole day. For these women it should be more appropriately labelled morning, noon and night sickness.

At its mildest, morning sickness simply causes a vague feeling of nausea, but many women have to cope with full-on vomiting which can at times be a little inconvenient to say the least! (My wife once doused our cat in her breakfast because she couldn't get to the toilet quickly enough.)

Don't be alarmed if you are one of those women suffering this level of vomiting; generally it does not affect the health of mother or baby. However, for a small number of women whose vomiting becomes relentless (a condition

Pregnancy is a magical time, but for many women it can at times feel more uncomfortable than enjoyable.

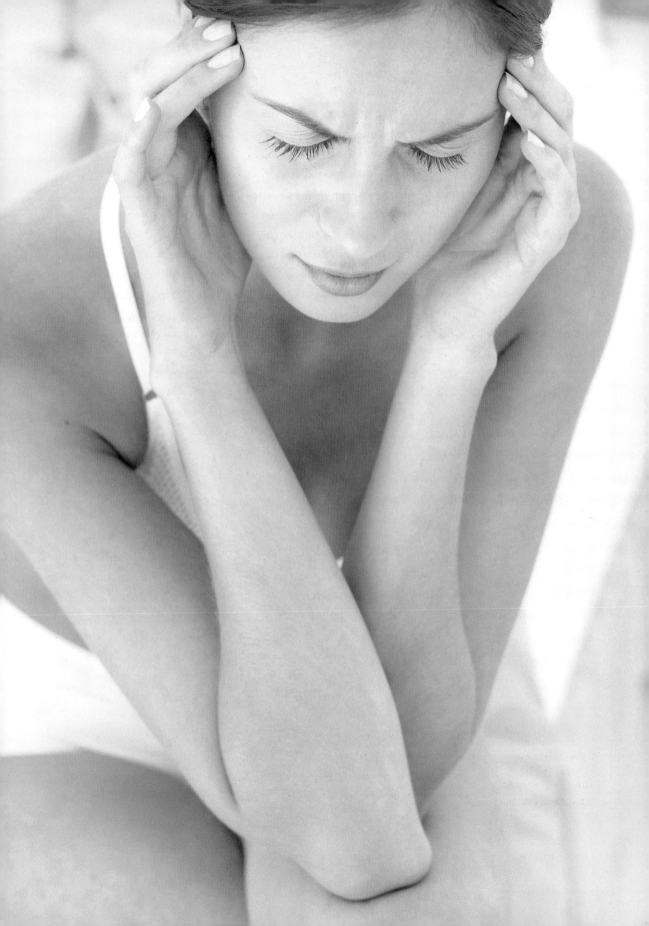

EASING MORNING SICKNESS

- Eat little and often – small frequent meals can help keep your blood sugar levels steady.
- Camomile tea can help – and it certainly won't hurt.
- If you are unfortunate enough to spend half your time being sick, make sure that you drink plenty of fluids to avoid dehydration.
- Avoid fatty foods as they take longer to digest, have strong nauseating aromas and are more unpleasant than most foods when revisited.
- Try eating bland foods like toast and dry biscuits.
- Ginger tea and biscuits have been found to keep nausea at bay.
- A number of medications (e.g. cyclizine and metoclopramide) are known to be safe in pregnancy and are prescribed by GPs if all else has failed.

There is also another drug that is available from your GP which is administered as an injection. The beauty of this method is that this drug will still work if your sickness is so bad that you can't even hold down pills.

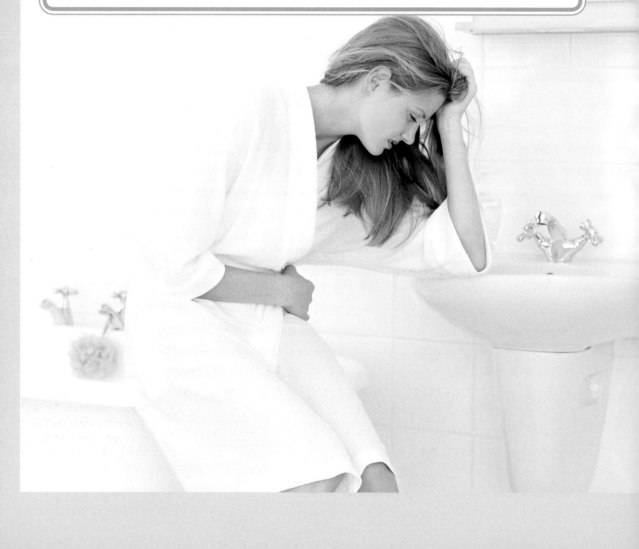

called hyperemesis gravidarum) there's a real risk of dehydration and weight loss. These women may need to be admitted to hospital where they will be put on an intravenous drip until things settle.

Over the years a long list of remedies have been touted as a cure for this problem; in fact there are probably as many proposed treatments as there are old wives to dream them up. (I Googled 331, 000 web pages on the subject.)

Of course, as we're all different, one woman's cure may either have no effect or even cause unwanted side effects in another, so it's advisable to try a variety of treatments before admitting defeat. (See box opposite.) Some advice is, however, simply unscientific twaddle.

But it's important to remember that if all else fails, time is often the great healer in this case and the symptoms are most likely to vanish by the end of the first trimester. If they don't or the sickness becomes disabling (trying to hold your lunch down while looking after your other children or functioning normally at work is no easy feat), the doctor can give you an injection to ease it, as a last resort.

Vaginal bleeding

Any sign of vaginal bleeding in early pregnancy will send a chill down the spine as it immediately sparks the fear that you are about to have a miscarriage. Although this is indeed one major cause of bleeding, it's reassuring to know that 50 per cent of the time a miscarriage isn't inevitable and you can still go on to have a normal pregnancy.

That does, unfortunately, mean that there is still a 50 per cent chance that you are having a miscarriage, which is obviously an extremely distressing thought. If accompanied by abdominal pain, the bleeding can also be a sign of an ectopic pregnancy. In all cases of bleeding you need to get in touch with your doctor straight away so that they can arrange an urgent ultrasound scan to find out what is happening.

Miscarriage

Miscarriage is extremely common and occurs in around one in six of all pregnancies (this risk increases as you get older). Technically this term covers a loss of a pregnancy right up until 24 weeks, but about 75 per cent of miscarriages will happen during the first trimester. Some will occur so early that you will have been completely unaware that you were even pregnant and they will simply seem like your next normal period.

Sadly, sickness isn't always confined to the morning, but the good news is that for most women it tends to lessen or disappear after the first trimester.

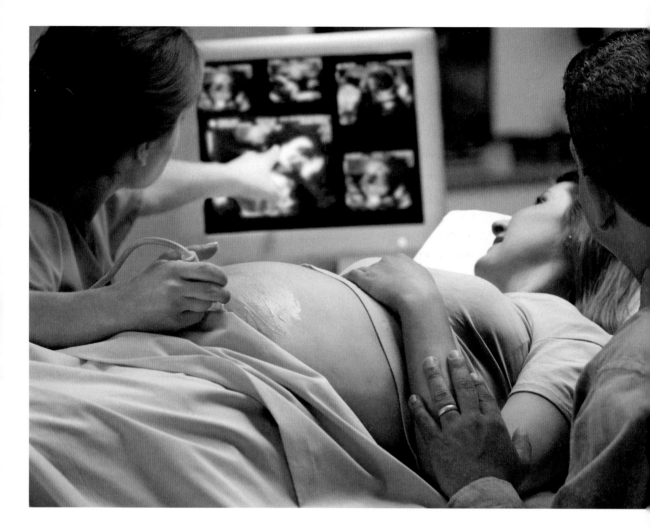

Scans have revolutionized the experience of being pregnant. They can bring good news as you see your baby for the first time, but sadly they can also detect ectopic pregnancies, miscarriages and problems with the baby.

The most important thing to remember if you have a miscarriage is that nothing you did brought it on and that there was nothing you could have done to have stopped it. Most of the time it happens because the embryo had a severe chromosomal abnormality, which means that it would never have developed properly and could not have survived. In effect, it's nature's way of dealing with a problem pregnancy.

Other less common causes of miscarriage include: hormonal problems (such as in polycystic ovary syndrome and out of control diabetes); an immune problem in which the mother's body rejects the baby; infections such as German measles (rubella) and cytomegalovirus; and problems with the shape of the womb (e.g. fibroids). At least half of all cases, very unhelpfully, have no identifiable cause.

If you see your doctor with bleeding, the chances are that they will refer you to the Early Pregnancy Assessment Unit at your nearest hospital where you will have a scan to check what's happening. Most of the time it's obvious what is going on and they will be able to tell straight away whether your baby is all right or whether this is, sadly, a miscarriage. Occasionally, if you are still quite early on in your pregnancy, it will not be so obvious and you will have to go back a week later to double check.

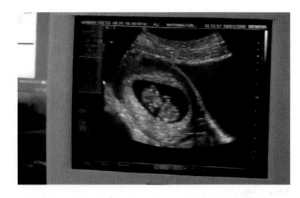

An ultrasound image will give you an amazing first glimpse of your baby – while still in the womb.

If the miscarriage is complete then the doctors will leave you be, but if some tissue has been left behind, you may need a small operation to prevent infection. This procedure is commonly known as a D and C (dilatation and curettage) and involves removing the contents and the lining of the womb under a general anaesthetic.

After a miscarriage it's important not to lose hope of carrying a baby – there's an excellent chance your next pregnancy will be fine. (In fact, even after three consecutive miscarriages there's still around a 70 per cent chance of succeeding at the fourth attempt.) Nevertheless, it's obviously an upsetting experience that can take some time to get over emotionally, so make sure you allow yourself time to grieve properly – with help from a support group if necessary – before trying again.

However, if you experience repeated miscarriages then you are likely to be referred to a specialist for investigation.

Ectopic pregnancy

This is a much rarer event which happens when an embryo loses its bearings and instead of implanting itself in the wall of the womb ends up elsewhere. These embryos most commonly settle in the fallopian tubes where they will start to cause symptoms of pain and perhaps vaginal bleeding.

An ectopic pregnancy can be extremely dangerous and can lead to life-threatening blood loss, so the embryo always needs to be removed. In an emergency situation, where the mother is collapsed and shocked, this is done surgically with an operation that warrants removal of the tube as well as its unwelcome contents (called a salpingectomy). However, many gynaecologists are now treating less severe cases with intramuscular injections of a drug called methotrexate, which avoids this drastic surgery.

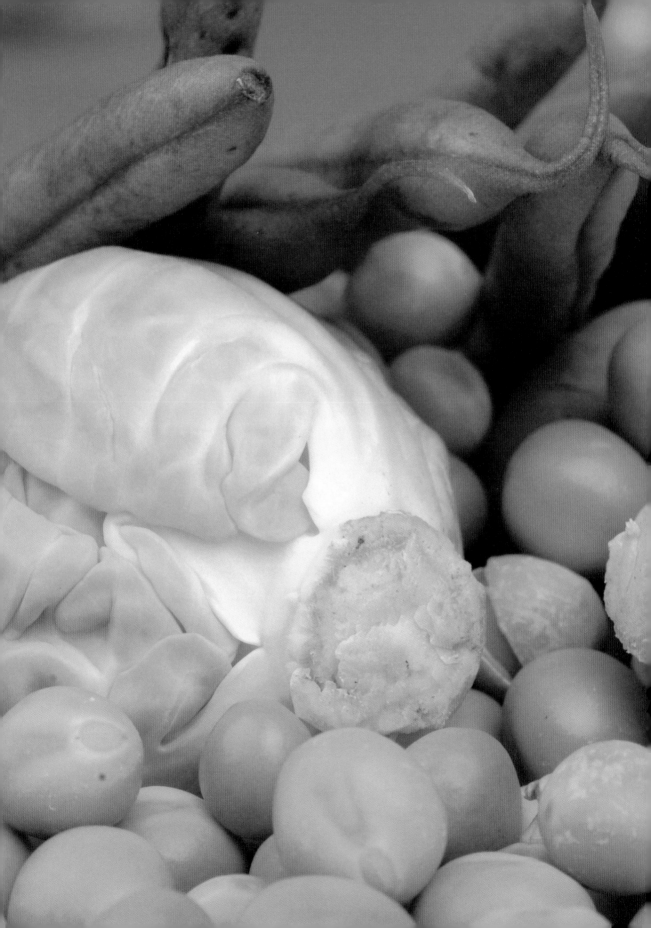

What's your baby up to in the first trimester?

While you're traipsing around between antenatal appointments trying to stay awake, avoiding wetting yourself and keeping the contents of your stomach down, your baby is going through the busiest time of its whole development.

It has just two weeks after fertilization to get itself from your fallopian tubes down to your womb and attach itself to the wall so it can switch off your periods and avoid being flushed away.

In general the embryo makes this journey with eight days to spare, and by day six it has already implanted in the wall of the uterus. Here it quickly begins to develop an early placenta, which in turn produces high levels of a hormone called human chorionic gonadotrophin (hCG) which overrides your hormone cycles, fending off your next period and, hopefully, the following eight.

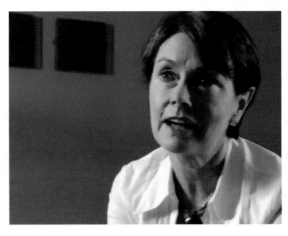

Expert Zita West advised all the couples featured on *Make Me a Baby* on the importance of diet for health and conception.

How your body changes

In the first trimester your body goes through huge changes to allow you to cope with the challenges of growing a baby.

Blood

The volume of your blood increases by around 40 per cent, and although the number of your red blood cells also goes up, this extra volume dilutes your blood causing a degree of anaemia. This is made worse by the extra demand your body has for iron, which your diet alone will find it hard to keep up with. You may well need to take iron tablets as a result, but remember that iron can be found naturally in many foods such as green vegetables, salad, red meat, boiled eggs, breakfast cereal and fish.

Blood circulation

Your heart also pumps larger volumes of blood each minute (cardiac output increases from 3.5 litres per minute to 6 litres per minute) to keep up with the extra demand on your body, and your blood vessels dilate to allow it to get to where it's needed more easily. This dilatation causes the lower blood pressure most women have during pregnancy.

Healthy eating is an important factor in anyone's diet, but munching on your greens is especially important for pregnant women to boost their stores of iron.

Respiratory

To meet the extra energy demands of building a baby, you will need to take on board up to 20 per cent more oxygen than usual (oxygen helps turns sugar in your body into energy). Hence you may well find yourself breathing more rapidly and feel short of breath when you exert yourself.

Blood clotting

Your blood clots much more easily when you are pregnant because the levels of proteins involved in clotting rise. This obviously helps stop bleeding at delivery from becoming torrential, but during the antenatal period it also increases your risk of having a deep vein thrombosis or pulmonary embolus (blood clot on the lungs).

Kidneys

Blood flow to the kidneys increases during pregnancy, which is what makes you want to pee more. There is also dilatation of the central chamber in the kidney (the pelvis) which makes urine drainage to the bladder slower and puts you at risk of urinary tract infections.

Skin and hair

The changes in your skin are more cosmetic than problematic. Your skin will generally become more pigmented, and often a dark line appears down the middle of your belly, called the linea nigra, and, of course, you can pick up every woman's nightmare – stretch marks. These marks often fade after delivery to virtually invisible silvery lines, but for many women they will always be a visible reminder of their pregnancy.

Your hair will also grow more during pregnancy, but these hairs will all be ready to drop out by the end of pregnancy – leading many woman to worry that they're going bald. The shedding of hair does stop, though, so rest assured you won't go bald and the hair does grow back again soon afterwards.

Gastrointestinal system

Everything in your gastrointestinal system slows down during pregnancy, presumably to allow more time for your body to absorb digested nutrients. It also means that they pass out more slowly too, so constipation can be a problem.

Those old chestnuts nausea and vomiting can also be rampant at this stage, as can acid reflux because of increased abdominal pressure pushing up on the

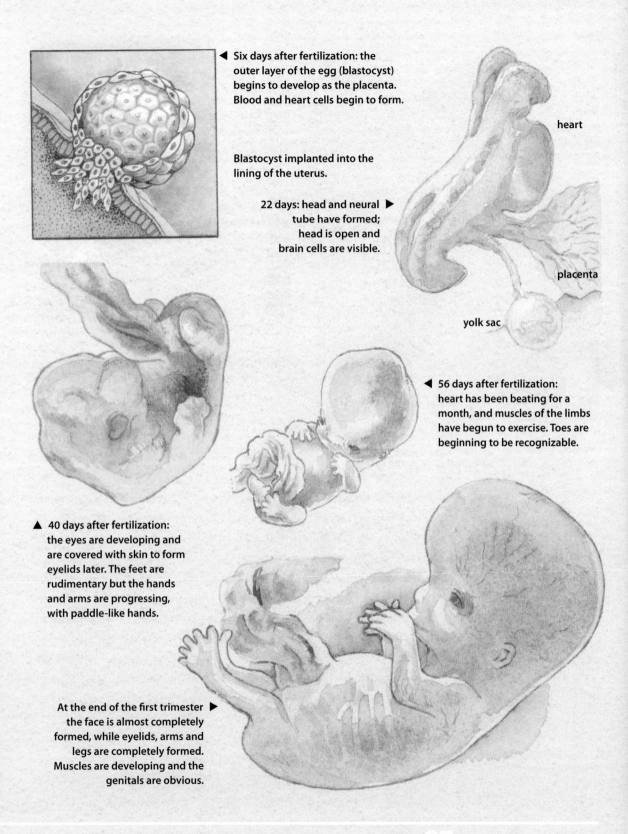

Six days after fertilization: the outer layer of the egg (blastocyst) begins to develop as the placenta. Blood and heart cells begin to form.

Blastocyst implanted into the lining of the uterus.

22 days: head and neural ▶ tube have formed; head is open and brain cells are visible.

heart

placenta

yolk sac

◀ 56 days after fertilization: heart has been beating for a month, and muscles of the limbs have begun to exercise. Toes are beginning to be recognizable.

▲ 40 days after fertilization: the eyes are developing and are covered with skin to form eyelids later. The feet are rudimentary but the hands and arms are progressing, with paddle-like hands.

At the end of the first trimester ▶ the face is almost completely formed, while eyelids, arms and legs are completely formed. Muscles are developing and the genitals are obvious.

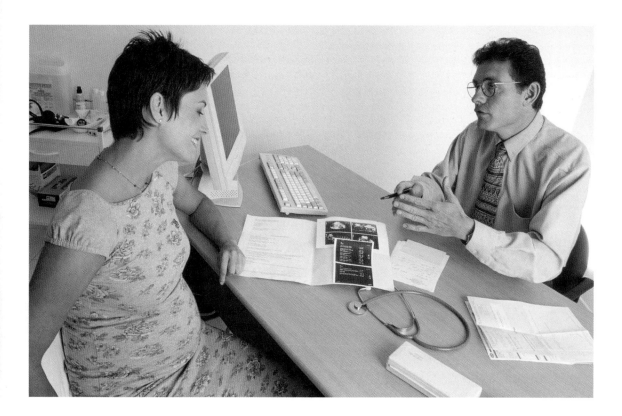

stomach. As your pregnancy continues, you may find yourself drinking antacids such as Gaviscon as if they were water.

Cravings for certain foods are also common, although we still don't really know why this happens. More nutritional foods make sense as these help to nourish your baby, but strange desires for things such as coal, chalk and soap are a little more of a mystery...

Finally, haemorrhoids (piles) can rear their ugly heads during pregnancy because of straining during constipation and the increased abdominal pressure. In order to ease the pain and bleeding these piles can cause it's important to keep yourself regular and try to keep your poo as soft as possible by drinking plenty of water and tucking into as much fruit and veg as you can stomach. If these tactics fail, then you might need to ask your doctor to take a peek at your tail end to assess the severity of your situation who might then prescribe something soothing.

Maternity benefits

You are entitled to a number of state-funded freebies during your pregnancy which include free prescriptions and free dental care, both of which will continue to be paid until your child's first birthday.

In order to claim these bennefits you will need a valid exemption certificate (the MAT B1 form), which your midwife will give you upto 20 weeks before your due date.

You are also entitled to maternity leave and maternity pay from your employer, or if you are self-employed or regularly paying National Insurance contributions you should also be entitled to Statutory Maternity Pay or maternity Allowance.

Maternity leave

You don't need to tell your employer that you're pregnant until 15 weeks before your due date, but it's always a good idea to let them know well in advance because it gives you protection against discrimination, the right to paid time off to go to antenatal appointments and any special health and safety protection that your job may require.

All pregnant women are allowed 26 weeks' maternity leave, and if you've been with the company for 26 weeks or more by the time you are 25 weeks pregnant then you are entitled to a further 26 weeks (unpaid) leave on top of that.

The earliest you can start your maternity leave is when you reach your 29th week of pregnancy, unless you agree otherwise with your employer.

Maternity pay

You are entitled to receive Statutory Maternity Pay if you have been employed for 26 weeks by the time you are 25 weeks pregnant and if you have been regularly paying National Insurance contributions. If you don't fall into this category, don't worry because all is not lost and you might still qualify for Maternity Allowance.

Your midwife can discuss the ins and outs of these benefits with you early on in your antenatal appointments, or see page 219 for who to contact for more advice and information on maternity benefits and entitlements.

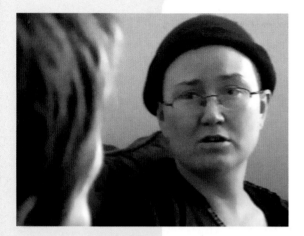

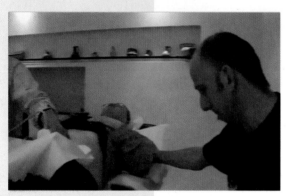

Susan and Alan had experienced previous miscarriages, so when they became pregnant again they paid to have an eight-week scan to reassure themselves that all was well with the baby.

Miscarriage

Experiencing a miscarriage is obviously one of the worst nightmares for any couple trying to have a baby, as Susan and Alan, who featured in *Make Me a Baby,* could testify; they had had far more than their fair share of this disappointment in this respect.

This couple have a two-year-old daughter called Marni, and then they decided to try for another. Although Susan became pregnant very quickly, they sadly had a miscarriage soon after. But they were determined to try again, and were delighted when Susan conceived again in the same year (2005) – this time with twins.

Sadly, tragedy was to strike once more, and at their 13-week scan they discovered that one of the foetuses had never really developed and the other had been lost at nine weeks. Susan had had no warning signs to suggest that she was miscarrying and in fact had continued to have all the symptoms that made her feel that she was still pregnant. It was a complete shock and they were both absolutely devastated.

But they were still very serious about having another baby and they wanted to start trying again as soon as possible, to help them move on from their grief. To improve their chances of keeping the next baby, they cut out caffeine and alcohol and started having sex every 36 hours during her fertile period, rather than every day, to ensure they didn't exhaust Alan's sperm supply.

Their efforts finally paid off at the start of 2006 when Susan had a positive pregnancy test. They were obviously extremely reluctant to celebrate at this point and Susan spent every waking moment fearing the worst. To ease the suspense, and to check that everything was ok, they paid to have an eight-week scan privately, and they went along to the hospital expecting to hear the worst. To their enormous relief, the scan was fine and they were able to see their baby's heartbeat.

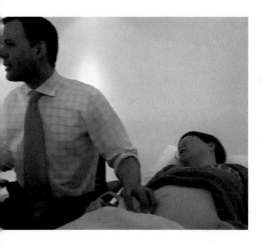

Despite the reassurance of this scan, Susan found it very difficult to feel positive and confident about the pregnancy. As a result she became incredibly depressed and even too fearful to leave the house in case something happened to the baby. So she began to spend all day sitting at home in their basement flat with little Marni, just waiting for what she saw as the inevitable unhappy ending of her pregnancy.

However, by the time Susan reached 20 weeks into her pregnancy she started to feel a little more positive, and having seen that her baby was developing normally at their twenty-week scan, both Susan and Alan began to enjoy the prospect of having a healthy baby. Finally they began to relax and look forward to getting their dreamed of brother or sister for Marni; a wish which became a happy reality for them in October 2006 when Susan gave birth to Cosi.

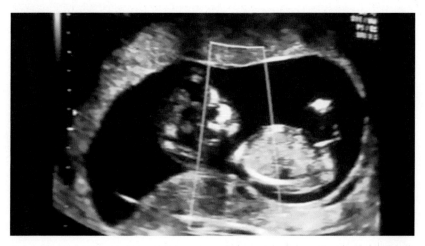

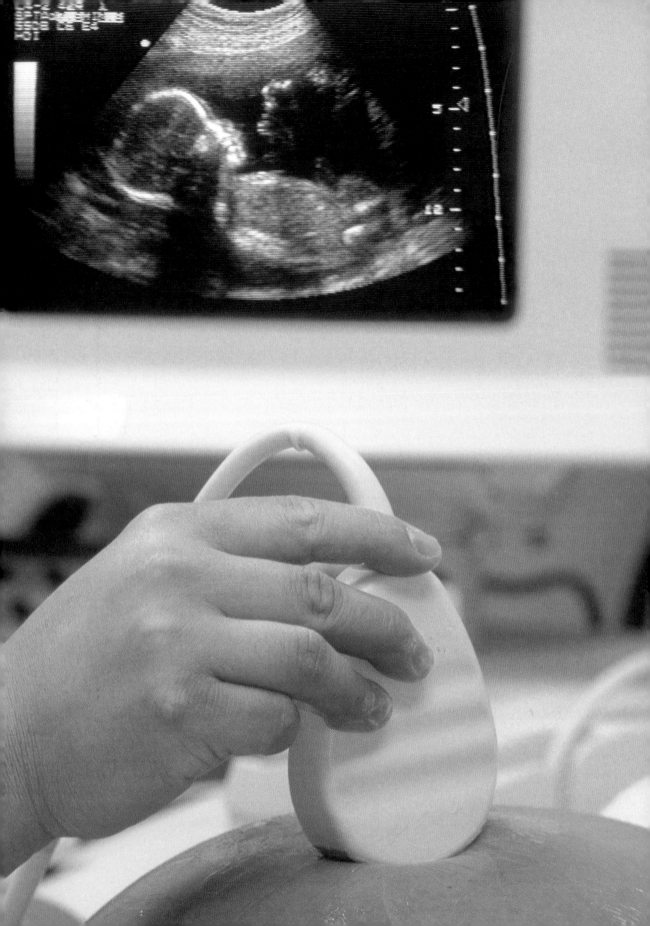

chapter 3

The second trimester

Many women utter an enormous sigh of relief as they cross the finishing line of the first trimester and head off into the second. Most will at last be able to wave goodbye to the horrors of morning sickness, and as their bodies get used to the idea of being pregnant, other symptoms will make their exits too.

The second trimester is the time when all the hassle seems worth it, when you feel your baby wriggling around inside you. You will finally have something to show for your troubles, too, as your belly expands and you find yourself going up a few waist sizes. Most importantly, though, it also means that the really risky days are behind you and the chance of a miscarriage is much less likely.

Trouble shoooting

However, the second trimester has some testing times of its own; quite literally in fact, as this is the stage of pregnancy when most of the tests looking for abnormalities are carried out. Two of the major problems that doctors are looking for at this stage of pregnancy are Down's syndrome and spina bifida, and many of the tests are performed to rule out these specific conditions.

Down's syndrome

Down's syndrome is a condition named after the person who identified it, rather than being an explanation of how it affects an individual. (Unlike yellow fever, for example, which does exactly what it says on the tin – it turns you yellow and raises your temperature.)

First described in 1866 by Dr John Langdon Down in an article in the *London Hospital Reports*, his paper's analysis of the babies in his care was the first to outline the features of this condition and to conclude that it was a congenital problem. However, it wasn't until much later, in 1958, that Professor Jérôme Lejeune and his team in France discovered that the condition occurred due to a baby having an extra chromosome – chromosome number 21.

The genetic code on chromosome 21 was one of the first to be identified by scientists involved in The Human Genome Project. It is believed to contain 329 individual genes, and it is the extra set of this chromosome that results in an abnormal translation of the genetic information which in turn causes the problems that babies with Down's syndrome can have.

Opposite: Coils of DNA combine to make the genes in our chromosomes.

Below: Down's syndrome occurs in babies that have an extra chromosome – chromosome number 21.

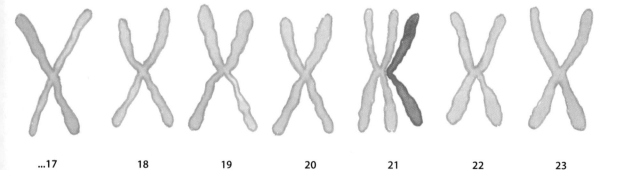

...17   18   19   20   21   22   23

THE SCIENCE OF DOWN'S SYNDROME

To explain the condition in simple terms, we have 23 pairs of chromosomes which are basically large molecules within our cells that contain our genetic material in the form of DNA (deoxyribonucleic acid). DNA molecules carry a code that can be translated into the blueprint for building all our bodily tissues and it is packaged into what are called genes – each of which code for different characteristics, for example, eye colour. These genes are then grouped on to our chromosomes – some of which contain literally thousands of them.

An analogy which will help with this is to imagine DNA molecules as being words; our genes are the page on which the words are written and a chromosome is the magazine in which those pages are stapled. Finally, a cell would be represented by a magazine rack where 46 pairs of these different magazines are shelved.

The chromosomes come in pairs because we get one from each of our parents; but this is where the pattern changes in Down's syndrome babies, and those who have this condition end up with one extra number 21 chromosome – a condition called trisomy. In most cases this duplication is believed to occur before conception when an egg, or more rarely a sperm, is made with two copies of this chromosome instead of one. This is a process known as meiotic nondisjunction.

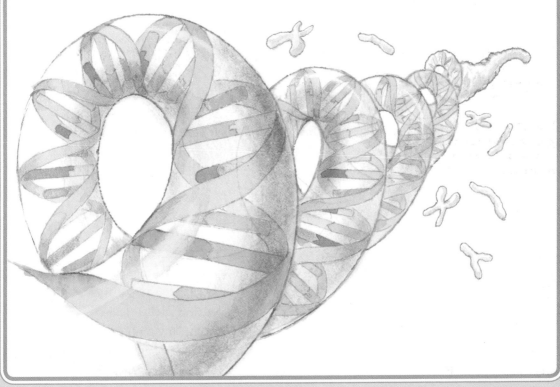

RISK OF DOWN'S SYNDROME	
Maternal age	**Risk**
Under 25	1:1500
30	1:900
35	1:380
40	1:110
44	1:35

In the UK, 1 in 1000 babies is born with Down's syndrome, but the risk of occurence is greater in older mums and increases with the age of the mother (see table, left).

Children with Down's syndrome share a number of common features which are present at birth:

- A flatter, more rounded face and flattening of the back of the head – known as brachycephaly.
- Eyes slant upwards and babies tend to have small mouths and large, often protruding, tongues.
- There are small folds of skin between the inner corner of the eye and the bridge of the nose (epicanthic folds), which make the eyes appear crossed.
- There may be white or yellow spots around the rim of the iris (coloured part of the eye) called Brushfield spots.
- The hair is straight and soft and the baby will have smaller ears.
- The hands may be broad with short fingers. (The little finger, in particular, may only have one joint instead of two.) There is often a wide space between the first and second toes.
- Poor muscle tone (hypotonia) in the arms, legs and neck; but this may improve with age.
- They may have just a single crease across the palm of the hand.
- They may suffer from heart defects – most commonly abnormal openings in the walls of the heart's chambers which prevent normal circulation.

As people with Down's syndrome get older, however, a number of further problems can also develop:

- Learning difficulties.
- Small stature – children with Down's tend to be shorter than average.
- Recurrent ear infections, which can cause hearing difficulties.
- Cataracts and squints, which can affect eyesight.
- A reduction in the amount of hormone released by the thyroid gland. This is a condition called hypothyroidism which can cause weight gain, constipation and depressed moods as a result of a slower metabolic rate.
- Alzheimer's disease tends to develop earlier in adults with Down's syndrome and occurs in 75 per cent of those people over the age of 60.
- Arthritis, diabetes, leukaemia and coeliac disease are also more common in those with Down's syndrome.

Of course, none of this sounds like good news (and on the face of it it makes pretty depressing reading), but over the past few decades medical and social care for children and adults with Down's syndrome has improved remarkably, and so has the potential quality of life for babies born with the condition.

Since 1983 the average life expectancy for people with Down's syndrome has increased from just 25 to 49. Where babies born in Dr John Down's day would have spent their short lives in institutions such as the one in which he worked, there are now great opportunities available to help those with the condition to play an active part in society and to reach their full potential: opportunities that they deserve as much as anyone else.

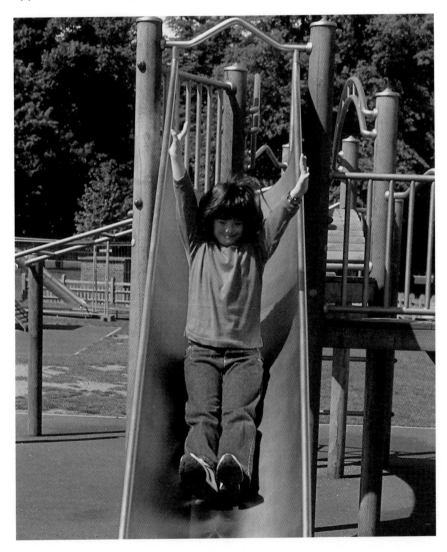

With so much information and support for Down's syndrome available today, children born with the condition can expect to play a full and active part in society.

Spina bifida

The medical term spina bifida literally means 'split spine'. This condition occurs between days 14 and 28 of a baby's development when one or more vertebrae (the bones which make up the spine) fail to form properly, leading to damage to the spinal cord. This occurs most commonly at around the level of the baby's waistline.

There are two main types of spina bifida:

- Spina bifida occulta, is thought to occur in up to 10 per cent of babies and is only noticeable by a small dimple or tuft of hair in the small of the back. The majority of babies with this type of spina bifida will experience no problems whatsoever.

- Spina bifida cystica is seen in two forms, namely meningocele and myelomeningocele. In meningocele there is a fluid-filled sac in the small of the back that contains the tissues which cover the spinal cord (meninges) and the cerebrospinal fluid which bathes it, both covered in a layer of skin. In myelomeningocele the sac also contains part of the spinal cord, which in this case tends to be damaged and not properly developed.

Many babies born with spina bifida also have hydrocephalus (which literally means water on the brain) because of abnormal circulation of the cerebrospinal fluid. This condition can cause increased pressure inside the skull, which as a result can enlarge beyond its normal size and cause damage to brain cells.

At the most serious end of the spectrum, problems with spinal cord development can lead to a condition called anencephaly, where the brain fails to develop properly – or even at all. Babies with anencephaly are either stillborn or die soon after birth.

Spina bifida is a condition that can be treated soon after birth with surgery, which will repair the defect. Hydrocephalus can also be treated by inserting a shunt (a tube made of silicone with one-way valves that direct the flow of cerebrospinal fluid) into the skull which will divert the extra fluid back into the bloodstream. Groundbreaking surgical techniques (see below) are also being developed which can treat spina bifida while the baby is still inside the womb.

Screening tests

Thanks to the wonders of modern technology there are a whole range of screening tests available to pregnant women – and most of them are free on the National Health Service. The purpose of these tests is to allow doctors to check your baby is developing as it should and to rule out the possibility of a number of chromosomal abnormalities.

By identifying problems at an early stage, doctors can anticipate any difficulties the baby might experience either at birth or in its early life. Some of these can even be corrected while the baby is still in the womb. These investigations also allow parents to be confident that all is well with the baby. But if it isn't, it gives them the opportunity to decide whether or not to continue with the pregnancy, or gives them time to make provisions for caring for a child with special needs.

> None of these tests are compulsory, and if you prefer your maternity experience to be more organic and natural and want to keep the medics at arm's length, you can. It's not against the law to refuse the tests and nobody will send the boys round to twist your arm.

Blood tests

Blood samples will continue to be taken in the second trimester for some simple and straightforward tests which will measure the levels of a number of chemical markers in your blood. The results of these tests are then used to calculate the risk of your baby having either Down's syndrome or spina bifida (see pages 74–8).

Blood samples are scanned for the following chemicals:

◊ Alpha-fetoprotein (AFP): made in a baby's liver, this protein can seep into the mother's circulation if there's a break in the baby's skin – as in spina bifida. The leakage produces a much higher level of AFP than expected in the amniotic fluid and in the mother's blood, which is picked up in these tests. Conversely, in Down's syndrome there is a lower level of AFP in the mother's blood than would be expected; why this happens isn't known.

◊ Human chorionic gonadotrophin (hCG): the level of this hormone is raised in mothers with Down's syndrome but, again, no-one yet knows why.

◊ Oestriol: the level of this hormone is also lower in the blood of those women carrying a baby with Down's syndrome.

Used alone the levels of these three chemicals have very little predictive value for Down's syndrome, but when combined in the triple test and analysed in conjunction with the mother's age, a risk value can be calculated.

I can't stress enough, though, that the result of the triple test is NOT diagnostic. If the figures reveal a high risk it does not mean your baby definitely has

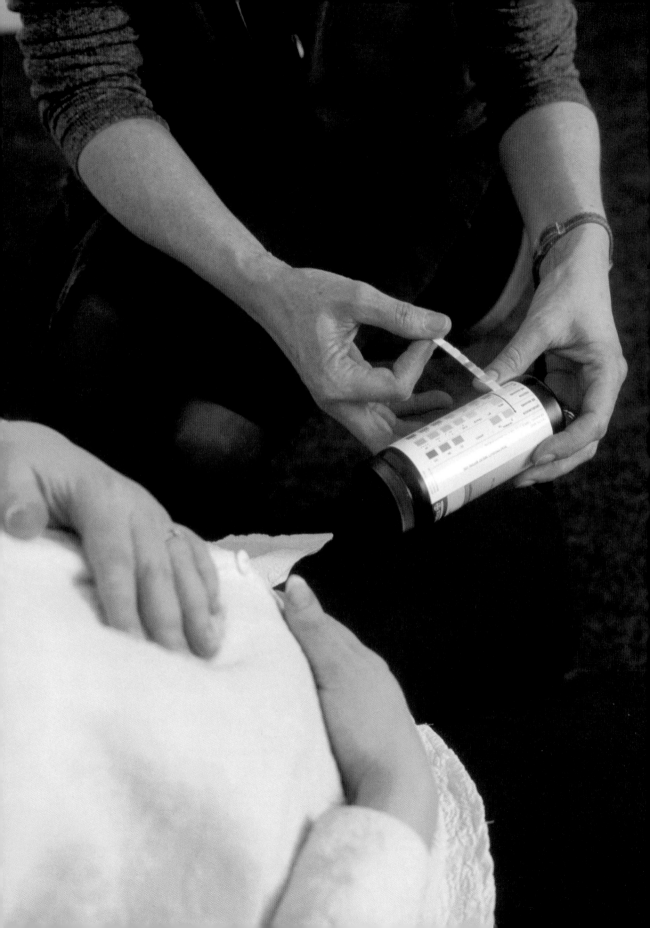

Down's syndrome (let's face it, a risk as high as 1 in 2 still means there's a 50 per cent chance of the baby being fine), and it just acts as a guide after which you and your doctor might decide you should have a more detailed test (such as an amniocentesis – see page 74).

However, this triple test carries the least risk for the baby and, unless you're scared of needles, won't do you any harm either, so many couples opt to go through with it.

Nuchal thickness scanning

This test is carried out in the form of an ultrasound scan so, like the blood tests above, it carries no risk to your baby. Usually this scan is carried out between 11 weeks and 13 weeks plus six days into your pregnancy and is able to pick up 80 per cent of babies with Down's syndrome. It is most often performed using a probe over the surface of your tummy, but in some cases a vaginal probe may be needed to get a more accurate image.

During this scan the specialist will be looking for a number of telltale signs which suggest that your baby has a higher risk of having Down's – but again this test is not 100 per cent accurate and only gives an indication that further tests may be needed.

Firstly, as the name of the test suggests, the nuchal thickness scan will concentrate on your baby's nuchal region (behind the neck). Because babies tend to lie on their backs when they are within the womb, fluid will build up in this area due to the effect of gravity (much as fluid builds up in your ankles if you sit still on a plane journey for hours on end). In Down's syndrome it's believed that the tissues are more stretchy because of a problem with the production of a tissue fibre called collagen, so there is more room in which this fluid can collect.

It is this increased nuchal thickness that the doctor is looking for when he or she performs this test; it's a useful measurement which can also flag up a number of other potential problems that a baby might have with its heart, kidneys and bowels.

Secondly, the specialist will check whether they can see a nasal bone (which can be missing in Down's syndrome), and finally they will analyse the image of your baby's heart to see if it has any leaky valves (a leaky tricuspid valve is another feature of Down's syndrome).

After all these observations have been made, your baby will be measured so as to give you an accurate idea of how far gone you are.

A familiar sight for all pregnant women at their antenatal appointments is a urine dipstick.

The results of all these tests are available to you immediately and will be explained to you in the course of the appointment, so there is no agonizing wait involved.

Amniocentesis

You will be offered an amniocentesis if your doctor feels that there may be a high risk of your baby having a condition such as Down's syndrome. This may be because you have a strong family history of chromosome problems; because you're an older mum; because you've had a high risk result in the triple test; or because your nuchal thickness scan has shown warning signs of the features of Down's.

An amniocentesis can be carried out from 15 weeks into your pregnancy onwards and involves an obstetrician poking a needle through your belly and into your womb to draw off some of the amniotic fluid around your baby. The fluid that is removed contains cells from the baby which can then be analysed for chromosome problems by the techies in the lab.

In order to avoid causing harm to your baby the procedure is carried out in sterile conditions and the needle is positioned under guidance from an ultrasound image. Despite this, and even in the very best hands available, the procedure still carries a 1 per cent chance of causing a miscarriage (even, and most distressingly, if the baby is normal).

Once the sample has been collected (which takes around ten minutes) it can take up to three weeks to get a result, which only adds to the anguish created by the whole experience. Nevertheless, if you've been scared to death by a previous test result, a normal result in this one is worth its weight in gold.

Chorionic Villus Sampling

This test is used to look for chromosome abnormalities, such as Down's, and for inherited disorders such as the lung condition cystic fibrosis. The beauty of this test is that it can be performed earlier than an amniocentesis (from 11 weeks onwards) and can give a result in a matter of days. It has the same level of accuracy but it does carry a slightly higher risk of miscarriage – of up to 3 per cent of all cases.

In this test, a sample of the placenta is removed for analysis, as this too has the same genetic make up as your baby. This sample material is collected using another big needle which can be inserted either through the belly wall again or through the neck of the womb (cervix) via your vagina. Again,

An amniocentesis is carried out under the watchful guidance of the ultrasound scanner.

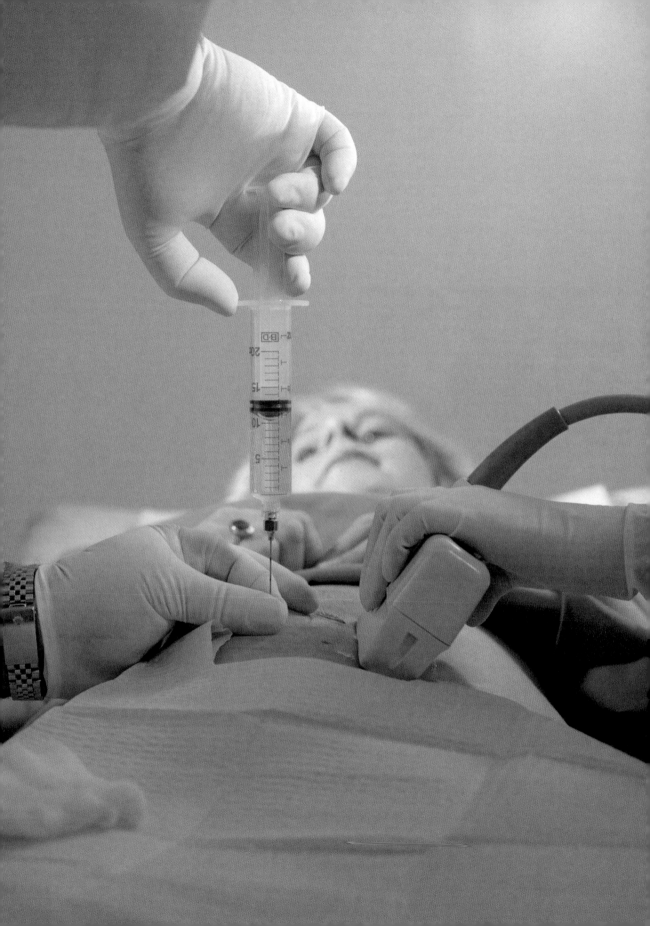

pinpoint accuracy is ensured by monitoring the whole process with an ultrasound scanner. The procedure only takes around 20 minutes and at the end of it the specialist will check the baby's heartbeat for you.

Given the inherent risks of the last two tests, most specialists will not advise that you have them unless your risk is at least as high as 1 in 300. Even then the odds of having a completely normal baby are heavily stacked in your favour, so it's very much down to you and your partner to decide whether those odds are worth the risk of having either test done.

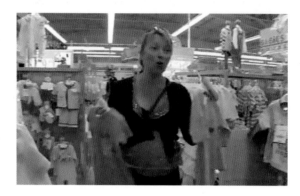

Will your twenty-week scan leave you buying clothes in pink or blue? And will you even want to know?

Twenty-week scan

This is the scan that most people are familiar with, as for some it is the one that supplies you with the first pictures of your little-uns for the family album. It's also the time when you can find out if it's a boy or a girl kicking away in there – if you don't have the patience to wait until it's born to decide what colour to paint the nursery. (Be prepared, though, that some maternity units may have a policy of not telling you, because it is a time-consuming exercise and they cannot guarantee accuracy anyway.)

You need to drink a lot of clear fluids before this scan so that you have a full bladder; this helps the scan operator to squeeze out any pockets of air between the womb and the bladder in order to get a better view. Of course, that does mean that if the scan takes a while it can get quite uncomfortable. But, aside from the desperate urge to run to the toilet, it's an otherwise harmless procedure and poses no risk whatsoever to either you or the baby.

So, once you are comfortably settled on the couch the sonographer will squeeze a dollop of freezing cold jelly on to your abdomen and begin to pick up images by moving a probe through this conductive gel across the surface of your skin. These images will appear in black and white on a screen in front of you and, despite looking like a blizzard on a dark night, once the specialist points out the different features of your baby to you it will all make sense. And it's a wonderful sight.

But it must be remembered that there is a serious medical reason for this scan (which doctors refer to as an 'anomaly' scan), and that is to check your baby for any obvious abnormalities. To that end the sonographer will study every organ from brain to bowel in great detail and make sure it looks just as it should do. The sonographer will also look at the way the heart is beating, the shape of the skeleton and even check your baby's facial features for signs of a cleft lip and palate.

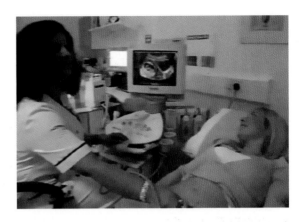

Once these observations have been made and noted, the baby's head and abdominal circumference will be measured, as well as its length from crown to rump, just to make sure that its growth is in step with its age. The amount of amniotic fluid in which it is swimming will also be calculated, because if there is too much then this gives a warning that there may be problems with the baby's gut, and if there is too little there could be something amiss with its kidneys.

The sonographer will be keen to get a good view of the placenta to make sure that it is well out of the way of your cervix and therefore not likely to complicate or prevent a vaginal delivery. However, if the placenta is found to be 'low-lying' at this early stage there is still a chance that it will move out of the way as your pregnancy progresses, but you might well be asked to return for a follow-up scan. If the placenta insists on sticking where it is – a condition called placenta praevia – then the doctors might suggest to you that your baby be delivered by Caesarean section.

And, of course, they will make sure you have one baby in there rather than two or more.

Twins

One of the most jaw-dropping moments for any parents-to-be is when they receive the news at their routine ultrasound scan that they've got two babies on the way, and not just the one that they were planning for. This experience tends to provoke a strong mix of emotions ranging from wild excitement to bowel-loosening fear; not only at the thought of having to look after two newborns rather than one, but also in anticipation of the cost of kitting them both out.

However, many women might already have had a suspicion that something out of the ordinary was going on way before 20 weeks, because the symptoms they've had in the first half of their pregnancy will have been far more severe than they had bargained for.

As a result they might feel much more tired than expected, because of the increased dilution of their blood and the consequent anaemia this causes, and morning sickness often becomes morning, noon and night sickness. In case that doesn't sound bad enough, there's more back pain, insomnia, indigestion and sorer breasts than in an expectant mother of one. Oh, and of course the belly is a little bit on the large side, scuppering any hope of parading around with a neat little bump framed in trendy maternity wear.

In the UK there is around a 1 in 80 chance of producing twins, but these odds do increase as the mother gets older, if there's a family history of multiple pregnancies or if the woman has undergone fertility treatment.

There are two common types of twin pregnancies: non-identical (dizygotic) and identical (monozygotic):

♦ Dizygotic twinning occurs when a woman releases two eggs instead of one during her monthly cycle and both are fertilized by her partner's sperm. As a result, each twin has its own placenta and membranes, and although they can both be the same sex, they will have different combinations of their parents' genes and so will not be identical.

♦ In monozygotic twinning there is only one egg and sperm, but soon after the embryo is formed it splits into two. If this occurs up to three days after fertilization, the embryos will have their own placentas and sacs, but if it occurs between four and seven days then they will share the same placenta but have separate sacs.

If the split occurs later still – between seven and fourteen days – then they will share a placenta and a sac. If twins form after two weeks – which is rare – there is an increased risk that they will be joined (so-called conjoined twins). Because monozygotic twins are formed from the same embryo they will be identical, regardless of whether they shared a placenta or not.

Carrying twins can also cause its own specific problems, beyond the logistics of looking after two babies.

Vanishing twin phenomenon is something that is more common than you might think. Although one in 80 pregnancies results in the birth of twins, it's believed that many more pregnancies actually start off this way but that very early on in the pregnancy one of the twins fails to develop and is reabsorbed by the mother.

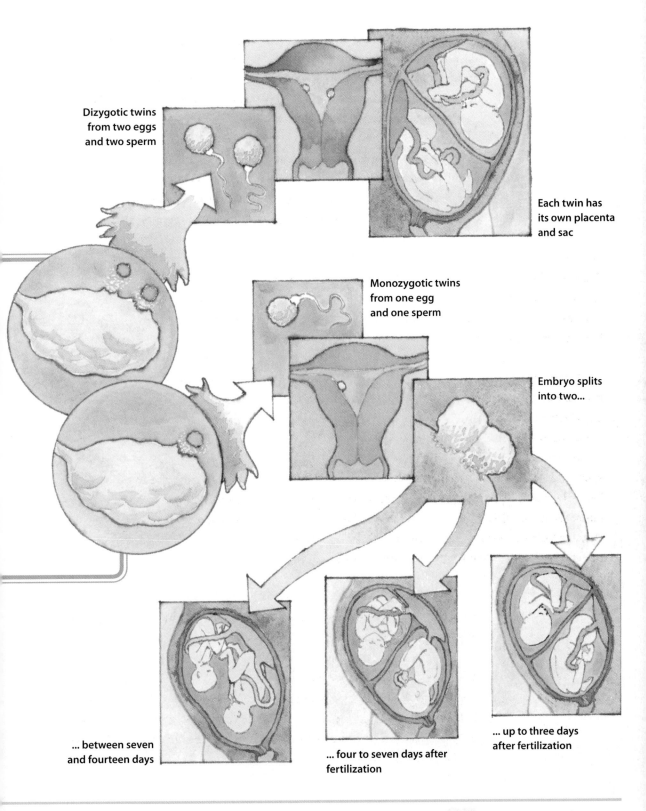

Dizygotic twins from two eggs and two sperm

Each twin has its own placenta and sac

Monozygotic twins from one egg and one sperm

Embryo splits into two...

... between seven and fourteen days

... four to seven days after fertilization

... up to three days after fertilization

The accuracy of scans is such that twin embryos and their sacs can be picked up by an ultrasound within six weeks of the start of a pregnancy. In studies that compare the number of twins seen on these early scans with the number that are actually born, it appears that this 'vanishing twin phenomenon' may happen in as many as one-third of twin pregnancies.

Twin-twin transfusion only occurs in pregnancies involving identical, monozygotic twins when there is a shared placenta and a link between the two babies' circulations. This can result in an unequal share in the blood supply, with one twin receiving too much and the other simply getting what's left. One twin may therefore become larger than the other, be at risk of developing heart failure and can also be surrounded by far too much amniotic fluid – a condition called polyhydramnios which can cause premature labour

Twin-twin transfusion makes identical twins look anything but, as one will be stealing all the goodness from the other.

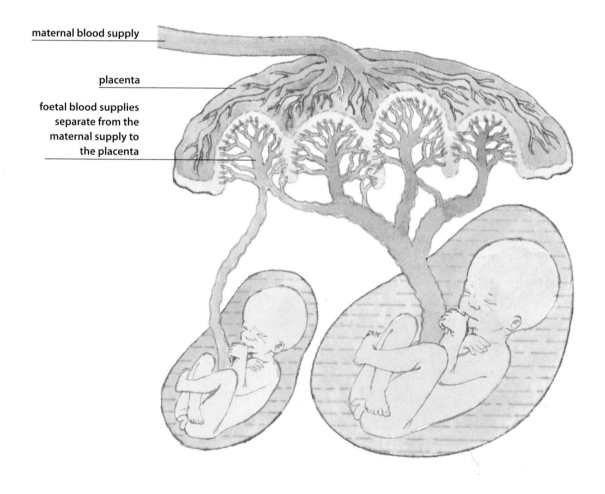

maternal blood supply

placenta

foetal blood supplies separate from the maternal supply to the placenta

and placental abruption when the waters break. The other twin's growth is consequently likely to be restricted and the baby could be at risk of becoming anaemic.

Treatment of this problem often simply involves removing excess amniotic fluid from around the larger baby, but in some hospitals the culprit blood vessels can be treated with lasers while the twins are still inside the womb. (See box about foetal surgery on page 91.)

Because there's a higher risk of problems during a twin pregnancy (see Chapter 4), antenatal care is rather more full-on for these expectant mothers than for a woman expecting just one baby. There will be more visits to doctors and midwives and, during the third trimester, many consultants offer scans at least every four weeks to monitor the babies' growth.

Antenatal infections

Aside from the previously mentioned common symptoms of pregnancy, an expectant mother can also find herself more vulnerable to the effects of a whole host of other illnesses and infections. Some of these are merely unpleasant or uncomfortable, but some can have a direct effect on the growth or development of your baby, or can even lead to miscarriage.

The most risky time for infections to cause serious problems or even result in the loss of a baby is in the first trimester and also at the beginning of the second; this can happen when the bugs which cause these infections pass into your baby's bloodstream across the placenta.

Here are some of the most commonly experienced infections, and a few tips on how to treat or avoid them.

Toxoplasmosis

This infection is caused by a parasite found in raw meat, unwashed fruit and cat poo. Around 70 per cent of women will not have had toxoplasmosis before pregnancy and although less than 1 per cent will pick it up while they are expecting, one-third of these will pass it on to their babies.

Unfortunately, although some women have a flu-like illness with a rash, fever and swollen lymph glands in the neck, many won't have any symptoms at all, so they won't know their babies are at risk. And the risks are big ones; infection in either the first or second trimesters has the potential to cause miscarriage, brain damage, epilepsy, deafness, blindness and growth problems.

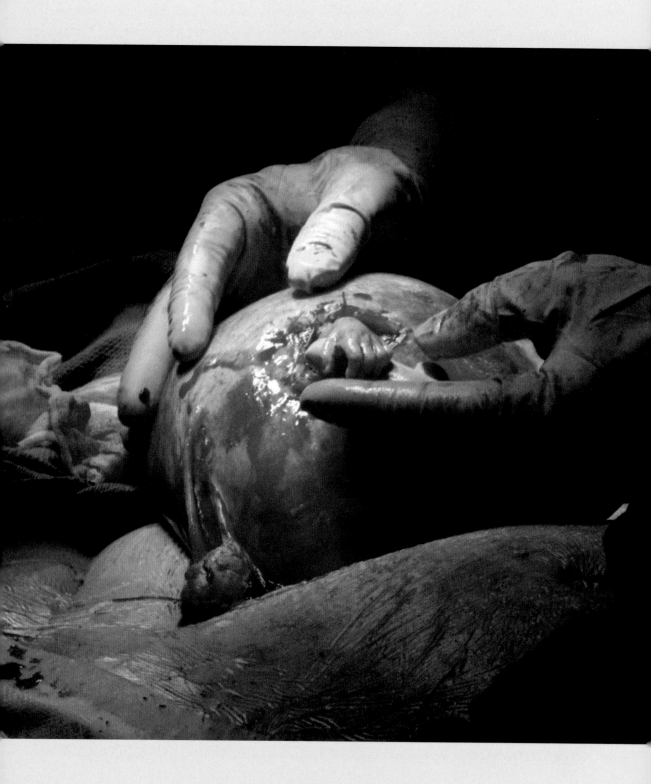

FOETAL SURGERY

Obstetricians have always prided themselves on having two patients to look after (the mother and the baby), rather than the mere one patient that the rest of us more humble doctors manage to treat. But until recently there hasn't been much that either medic could do for the baby while it was still in the womb, and what little they could do revolved around whacking doses of drugs into the mother and letting the placenta do the hard work of passing them on to her child.

However, in the past 20 years doctors in Britain and in the United States have been developing techniques that allow them to operate on a baby while it's still in the womb.

It sounds a bit far fetched, and a little like something out of science fiction rather than science fact, but thanks to these pioneers it's now possible to treat a foetus that might otherwise have had a poor chance of survival, or whose condition may be much more difficult to treat once they're born.

The process is, of course, fraught with dangers – not least the risk of setting off a miscarriage or harming the baby – but for some conditions there has been a fair amount of success. Such surgery has most commonly been performed using a procedure called a hysterotomy; where the operation is carried out by making a hole directly in the wall of the womb which is big enough for the surgeon to get their fingers into. However, science marches on and doctors are now developing keyhole techniques with an instrument called a fetoscope. This probe only needs the surgeon to make a 3–4 mm hole in the abdominal wall and uterus, and with its fibreoptic camera it allows surgeons to see exactly what they're doing.

Currently this type of surgery is being used to treat such problems as:

◊ Congenital diaphragmatic hernia – where there is a hole in the diaphragm (the muscle sheet between the chest and the abdomen) and so the guts and abdominal organs can spill up into the chest and hamper lung development.

◊ Twin-twin transfusion – where lasers are used in conjunction with fetoscopy to separate the blood vessels connecting a pair of twins.

◊ Spina bifida – there is doubt about the safety of this type of surgery as spina bifida isn't a life-threatening condition and the surgery can cause the baby to be lost. The jury is therefore still out.

Although these techniques are beginning to be used around the world in specialist centres, your GP is unlikely to be able to refer you to your local hospital for them for some time to come.

During a pioneering operation on an unborn child, the baby reaches out to touch the surgeon's hand.

Thankfully, there are many things you can do to avoid this infection:

- Eat well-cooked meat.
- Wash all fruit and vegetables before eating them.
- Wear gloves when gardening and wash your hands afterwards in case cats have been using your flowerbeds as a toilet.
- Get someone else to empty a soiled cat-litter tray for you, or if you have to do it yourself, always wear gloves.

Cytomegalovirus

This virus is a member of the herpes family and is a rare cause of deafness and cerebral palsy in babies. Most women will already have had cytomegalovirus before without knowing it and so will be immune by the time they are pregnant – and even those who do pick it up only have a 40 per cent chance of passing it on to their babies, of whom 90 per cent will be absolutely fine.

Listeria

This is a pretty rare bacterial infection which can be passed on through various foods, most notably soft ripe cheese (e.g. brie, blue cheeses and camembert), seafood, ready-to-eat (e.g. microwave) meals that haven't been cooked and heated through properly, pâtés, soft ice-cream and unpasteurized dairy products.

All of these foods should therefore be avoided like the plague in pregnancy – as should contact with live sheep and lambs, which can also carry it.

Listeria only tends to cause diarrhoea and vomiting in expectant mums, but, more worryingly, it can also cause miscarriage, stillbirth and encephalitis (infection around the brain) in their babies.

Rubella (German measles)

Infection with this virus can cause cataracts, deafness, cerebral palsy and various degrees of mental retardation in the unborn baby; hence all women have a blood test at their booking appointment to check for immunity to rubella.

Parvovirus

This virus is spread by droplets in the air from coughing or sneezing and causes a disease in children called Erythema infectiosum – more commonly known as slapped cheek syndrome because of the rosy red rash that appears on the face. In adults, parvovirus causes a fever with joint aches and pains and a lacy red rash on the arms, legs and trunk.

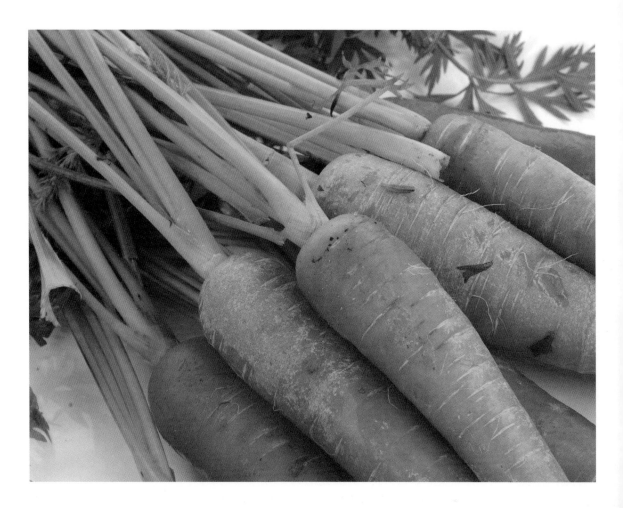

If this virus reaches the baby in the first 20 weeks of pregnancy then there's the risk of miscarriage or severe anaemia. Infection after that is much less of a problem.

Chicken pox

Most people catch chicken pox as children, but those who've slipped through the net and aren't immune as adults can pass it on to their babies if they get it. Thankfully there's less than a 1 per cent chance it will cause problems in the first trimester or the second, but if it does then it can be pretty serious and include limb and nervous system damage.

In the third trimester (particularly from week 36 onwards), up to 50 per cent of babies can get chicken pox from infected mothers, half of whom will develop symptoms of the virus. At this stage of pregnancy this can be fatal, so

To keep yourself and your baby healthy and out of harm's way, wash all fruit and veg before eating them – especially if you buy organic veg fresh from the ground.

babies born with chicken pox will receive intensive treatment with antiviral drugs and anti chicken pox immunoglobulin.

Medical conditions and pregnancy

If you have a pre-existing medical condition, such as asthma, epilepsy or diabetes, you are likely to receive special attention from your doctor and midwife during the antenatal period. They will carefully monitor your pregnancy to ensure that any problems these diseases might cause can be nipped in the bud before they do you or your baby any harm.

Asthma

Asthma affects the small airways (lung tubes); these carry oxygen in and out of the lungs by making them narrower. This reduction of the airways causes a number of symptoms, most notably shortness of breath, a persistent cough and a wheezy sound as air rushes through the tubes (much like wind in a tunnel). All of these can be extremely disabling, as they make sufferers quite literally run out of puff.

There are loads of different triggers for asthma – such as pollution, viruses, cat and dog hair, and even cold weather – which make these tubes tighten up and therefore set off a reaction. The good news is that asthma is very treatable. A sufferer will be prescribed an inhaler (some people call them puffers) which uses drugs that are breathed directly into the lungs themselves to open up the airways. However, an asthmatic may need steroid tablets (which reduce inflammation in the airways) and oxygen to get through a serious attack.

Around 5 per cent of pregnant women have asthma, and if you are one of them then the good news is that your symptoms are likely to get better during your pregnancy. All asthma treatments (such as ventolin, becotide or serevent inhalers) are known to be safe during pregnancy and breastfeeding, and there is no evidence that they cause birth defects or problems at either time.

If, however, you have bad asthma that requires you to take steroid tablets (prednisolone) then you may need to be given intravenous steroids (treatment through a drip) if you are suffering during labour.

Epilepsy

In epilepsy the normal electrical signals in the brain become chaotic, which leads to fits or seizures. The effect that these fits have on a person depends upon which part of the brain is affected. So if they occur in only a small part of the brain (a partial seizure) they may just cause twitching of, say, a hand or an arm, but if the whole brain is involved (generalized seizures) a person can lose consciousness, fall to the floor and have a convulsion.

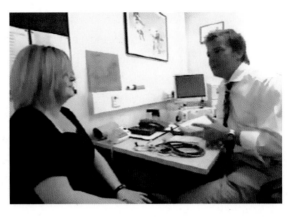

Epilepsy can't be cured with drugs but a number have been developed (called anticonvulsants) which can stabilize the brain's electrical activity and so cut down the number of seizures a person suffers. Unfortunately they're rarely 100 per cent effective, and most of them also have some potentially grotty side effects. In pregnancy these drugs can lead to an increased risk of miscarriage in the first trimester and to birth defects (such as cleft lip and palate).

On the up side, fit frequency doesn't necessarily increase in pregnancy but drug doses will need to be adjusted to take into account the impact of increased blood volume, as this dilutes the drug level and so cuts down its effectiveness.

Regular appointments during pregnancy are important for your doctor to keep an eye on any pre-existing medical conditions you might have.

If you suffer with epilepsy you will also need to take a higher dose of folic acid (5 milligrams instead of 400 micrograms) than other pregnant women, to protect against the greater chance of neural tube defects that these drugs can produce – such as anencephaly and spina bifida. You will also be referred to a neurologist (if you don't already have one) who will prescribe the right drug dose for you, and an obstetrician to monitor your baby's development.

But despite the risks, it's important to remember that there is a 90 per cent chance of having a trouble-free pregnancy and a completely healthy baby.

Diabetes

Unlike the previous two conditions, which you tend to have before you become pregnant, it's possible to develop diabetes while you are pregnant.

Diabetes is a condition in which the body has problems controlling the level of sugar (glucose) in the blood. In those people who develop it when they are children (called type-1 diabetes), this usually occurs because they don't make enough of a hormone called insulin, whose job it is to keep blood sugar levels steady. In older people diabetes often develops because their body's receptors for insulin become less sensitive (type-2 diabetes), and this is most commonly caused by obesity.

Either way, diabetics will be prone to huge variations in sugar level which in the short term can cause acute attacks of either hyperglycaemia – very high blood sugar – or hypoglycaemia – which is the opposite. Both of these can result in coma and even death.

But the longer term complications are pretty grim too. Poorly controlled blood sugar can affect almost every system in the body and can lead to blindness, loss of nerve sensation in the hands and feet, an increased risk of heart disease and stroke, and a shorter life expectancy.

Thankfully diabetes can be treated either by a combination of drugs and diet to keep the levels steady, or by replacing the lack of natural bodily insulin with daily insulin injections. Sufferers require regular check-ups and must keep an eye on their blood sugar levels every day. But it's worth the effort, because control can go a long way to stave off the potential horrors listed above.

In the first trimester of pregnancy, poor blood sugar control in women with pre-existing diabetes also increases the risk of a number of foetal problems, such as abnormal development of the heart, kidneys, brain and spinal cord. This is why they need particularly close monitoring.

But diabetes can also develop for the first time during pregnancy because many of the natural pregnancy hormones push up the level of blood sugar. Most of the time this is matched by an increased production of insulin and no harm is done, but if a woman's insulin fails to keep pace with its extra workload sugar levels will stay permanently high and a temporary condition called gestational diabetes will develop. (This type of the condition will be reversed once the baby is born and the hormone levels go back to normal.)

However, this form of diabetes can be bad news for babies because their own blood sugar level will rise when glucose crosses the placenta from their mothers. As a consequence these babies may well be bigger (which can make delivery more difficult), are more likely to be breech, or can be at risk of premature labour and, sadly, intrauterine death.

At delivery, babies born to diabetic mothers can also have dangerously low blood sugar levels and be at greater risk of having lung and therefore breathing problems.

These potential problems are just the tip of a rather depressing iceberg for both mother and baby, so special care is essential for mothers diagnosed with diabetes in order to address the condition as early in pregnancy as possible. Your blood sugar level will be checked whenever you present your midwife with a urine sample, and if the level on the dipstick gives cause for concern

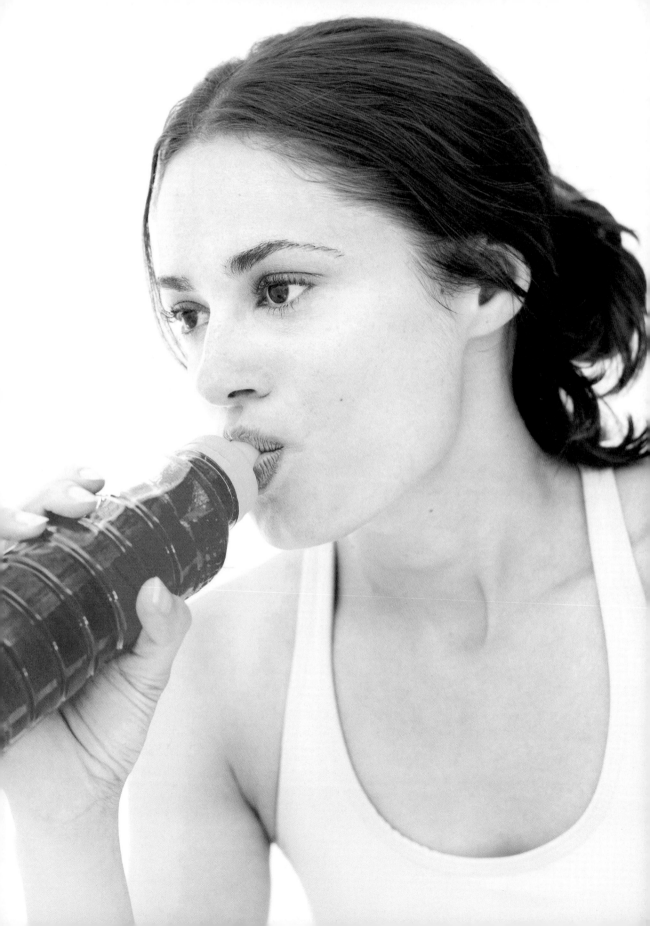

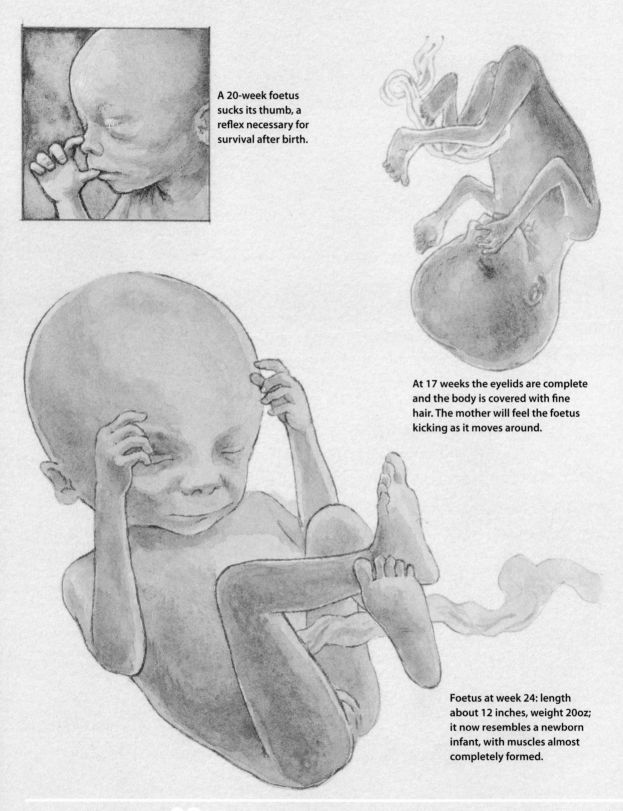

A 20-week foetus sucks its thumb, a reflex necessary for survival after birth.

At 17 weeks the eyelids are complete and the body is covered with fine hair. The mother will feel the foetus kicking as it moves around.

Foetus at week 24: length about 12 inches, weight 20oz; it now resembles a newborn infant, with muscles almost completely formed.

you're likely to be asked to take a blood test to get a more accurate idea of your sugar level.

You may also be asked to undertake a glucose tolerance test. With this test the midwife will be able to see just how well your body deals with a big (75g) dose of glucose in the form of a 350 ml bottle of Lucozade. They will take two blood samples: one at the start after fasting overnight (nothing to eat or drink but water from midnight the night before) to get a baseline level, and a second one two hours after your glucose drink.

GLUCOSE TOLERANCE TEST

Glucose level (mmol/l)	Fasting	2 hours
Normal	<7.0	<7.0
Impaired	<7.0	7.8 –11.1
Diabetes	>7.0	>11.1

If everything's working normally, after two hours the test should produce a normal glucose reading, but if you have gestational diabetes then the level will be high.

A third possible outcome is that you are diagnosed with impaired glucose tolerance because, although your two-hour level wasn't sufficiently high enough to meet the criteria of diabetes, it was higher than normal (see box).

Treatment of gestational diabetes is the same as for the pre-pregnancy condition and involves injections of insulin to keep the sugar level within the normal range. In impaired glucose tolerance, changes to a low-sugar diet may be enough to control things, but a proportion of women might still end up on insulin if the sugar level creeps up.

And now for some good news!

Having started this chapter by saying that most women breathe a sigh of relief when they reach the second trimester, much of what's been said since makes it sound more like the trimester from hell.

But it isn't – honest – it's just that doctors are used to spending their time hunting disease and not dealing with people who are healthy. Experience dictates that whenever our bodies are given the chance, they will let us down – hence all the tests and appointments and the infamous pots full of wee.

Sadly, this chapter has shown that at times this theory is correct and that for some women pregnancy can be fraught with problems and potential heartache. But, I can't emphasize enough that for the overwhelming majority of women things go well – medical paranoia can be completely unfounded and intervention can be surplus to requirements.

In the second trimester your baby's development starts to become more specialized.

By and large the second trimester is a great time for both mother and baby. In fact, for your baby it is one of the busiest times of their young lives – a developmental rollercoaster – as they change from what looks like a tadpole in the first trimester into a mini human complete with fully functioning organs, facial features and the ability to career around inside you using their umbilical cord as a bungee rope. This is the time when you can start to feel that wonderful sensation of your offspring kicking the living daylights out of your insides.

Studies have also shown that in the second trimester babies are already beginning to develop memory. In an experiment published in the medical journal *The Lancet*, in 1988, babies whose mothers had watched the Australian soap opera *Neighbours* while they were in the womb became quiet and contented in the first few weeks of life when they heard the theme tune on television, demonstrating that even at that early stage of development they were capable of learning. (Although hopefully developing a love of soaps won't prove to be the pinnacle of their intellectual achievements.)

Hyperemesis gravidarum

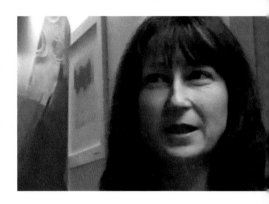

Hyperemesis gravidarum is the Latin name for a condition which causes profuse and uncontrollable vomiting during pregnancy. It is the mother of all cases of morning sickness and knocks most women's experiences of feeling a bit queasy in the first few weeks of pregnancy into a cocked hat.

Fortunately, this condition only affects up to 1 per cent of all pregnant women, and although there are a number of theories about what might cause it, nobody is really sure. The main suspects, however, are hormones (especially high levels of hCG), and genetics (it tends to run in families). It is also likely to affect women who've experienced it in a previous pregnancy.

Barbara was one such unlucky woman. She and her husband Andy already had a three-year-old boy called Joshua, and Barbara had been severely sick for the first half of that pregnancy. Sadly, her experiences in her second pregnancy turned out to be no different.

Barbara was physically sick a number of times throughout every day of the first 18 weeks: most foods and drinks (even water) would make her vomit and there

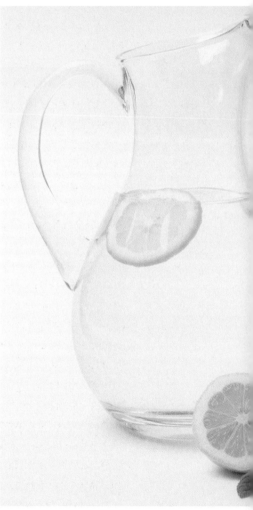

were even some smells which would immediately send her dashing to put her head down the toilet. As a result she was completely incapable of going into work and, more worryingly for the baby, she wasn't gaining any weight. Eventually the persistent vomiting caused her weight to plummet and she was admitted to hospital. There the doctors put her on an intravenous drip to rehydrate her and she was kept in and carefully monitored until her vomiting stopped.

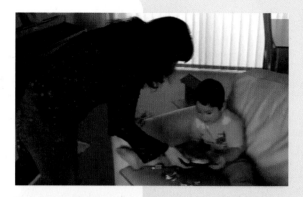

For all women with hyperemesis gravidarum, dehydration is the greatest danger. However, the doctor is able to spot the warning signs of this as it often shows itself first as a drop in the production of urine. Women therefore don't need a pee as often as they usually would and even then when they do produce it is, quite literally, nothing but small volumes of very dark yellow urine.

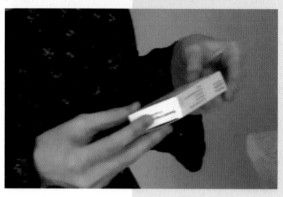

Hyperemesis gravidarum is a miserable condition that afflicts a tiny minority of unlucky pregnant women, such as Barbara. The constant sickness can make ordinary activities such as going to work and looking after other children a real challenge.

In severe cases of this condition the mouth and skin can become very dry, and when people with extreme dehydration cry they even find that they have too little fluid to produce tears. In all of these cases medical attention is needed as a matter of priority, but the good news is that the situation can easily be corrected by the woman being given fluids through a drip.

Fortunately, Barbara's symptoms did eventually settle and her pregnancy continued without any further difficulties. And later she and Andy were rewarded with a very healthy little girl called Molly Mae.

(If you are suffering extreme morning sickness, contact the hyperemesis gravidarum awareness group called Blooming Awful, at www.hyperemesis.org.uk.)

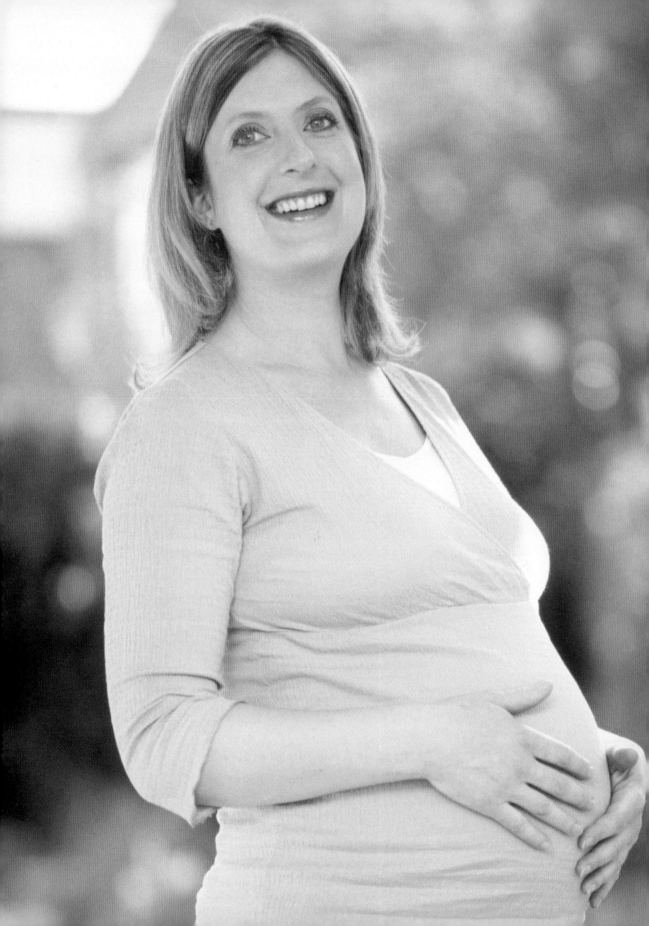

chapter 4

The third trimester

So here it is: the final stretch, the home run, the last lap of your pregnancy. With two-thirds down and just one more to go you're so close to the end that not only can you see the finish line ahead of you, you can virtually smell your baby's first nappy.

But your bun's not ready to come out of the oven just yet; there's still some very important cooking to be done in the thirteen weeks that make up the third trimester. And, boy, will you know about it – because as your baby gets bigger so, by default, will you.

Many women describe this as the most uncomfortable period of the whole nine months, when even the most basic manoeuvres – such as standing and sitting – become a struggle. And as for walking, well there's a reason why women at this stage of pregnancy waddle everywhere with their feet wide apart, elbows bent, hands pressed into the curve of the small of the back sporting a pained expression on their faces: that's because it's physically impossible to do it any other way. So for the next couple of months it's more than likely that a career of gliding gracefully down a catwalk, or anywhere else for that matter, is completely out of the question.

However, this stage of the game also brings great excitement – albeit tinged with some trepidation. You're going to have a baby – and soon – so there's a nursery to decorate, clothes and kit to buy, a name to decide on and a birth plan to write. So while you'll feel like putting your feet up more than ever now, unless you've been super organized before this point, there's likely to be less time for you to do so.

What's your baby up to in the third trimester?

In these final weeks your baby will really start to pile on the pounds, because now it is beginning to store fat to help it maintain its body temperature once it hits the outside world. In fact, during this trimester your baby will gain around half a pound per week and its weight will shoot up from around 4lbs (1.8kg) to anything up to 10lbs (4.5kg) – for those poor unfortunate women who specialize in squeezing out whoppers. (If you are Ms Average, however, you'll be pleased to know that your baby is more likely to weigh in at a slightly less eye-watering 7.5–8lbs (3.5kg).)

By 28 weeks your baby's eyes will be opening and closing and it will be able to see and hear. Eye colour will also have been determined by this point; however, some babies might be born with blue eyes but then undergo a colour change during the first weeks after birth.

The lungs are not yet mature at this point, although your baby will go through some of the motions of breathing as it makes rhythmic ▶

During the seventh month your baby's eyes will open and shut. They will put on about another 4lbs and their internal organs start to prepare themselves for life outside the womb..

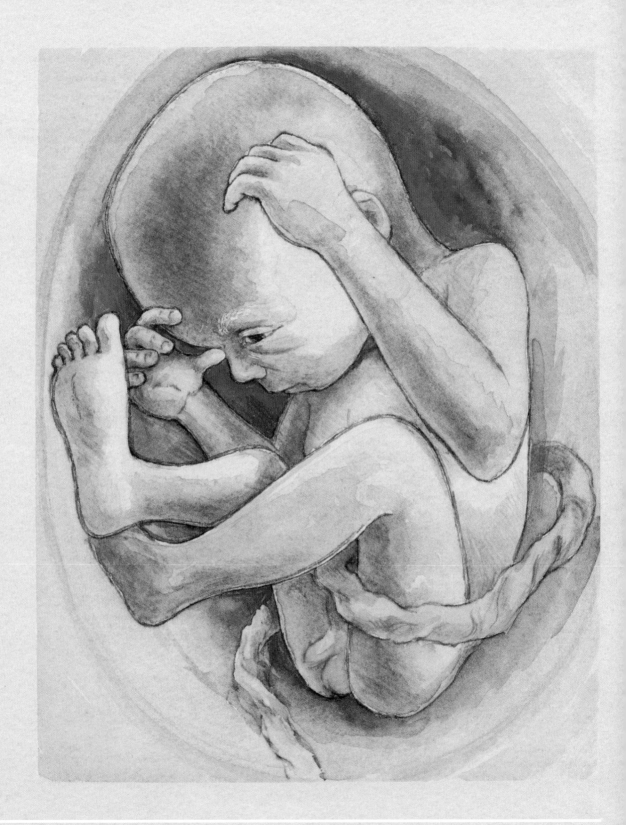

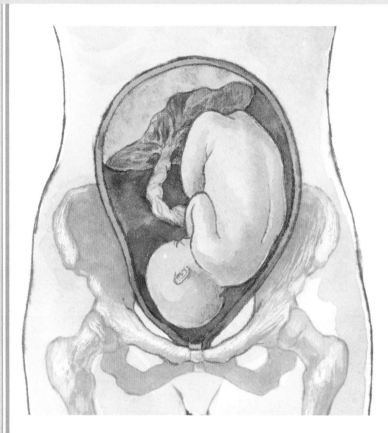

At around 36 weeks in first-time mothers, the baby's head drops into the pelvis as it starts to engage ready for delivery.

movements of its diaphragm. These can at times lead to it developing hiccups which, expectant mothers tell me, can feel quite weird.

The kidneys have a little way to go as well but, by and large, in the first few weeks of this trimester your baby's organs are ready to perform their various jobs once the umbilical cord is cut and you cease to do it all for them. **At around 31 weeks**, baby boys will experience their testicles starting their journey from the kidney area, where they have been developing, down towards the scrotum. If your baby is a girl, then her clitoris will start to become prominent at around this time too.

By about week 33 your baby will start to get into position for delivery, with its head moving down into your pelvis. As your baby grows there's less room for manoeuvre, so by now if it's not pointing in the right direction you may have to prepare yourself for having a breech baby (see page 158). However, if your baby hasn't lost its bearings then you can expect its head to drop firmly into the pelvis by around 36 weeks in a process called 'engagement'. As it does so it will generally point downwards (its face looks towards your backside), again to help with delivery. Some babies might choose to face the other way, which can cause problems at delivery.

As the third trimester progresses, your baby will sleep for about half an hour at a time but when it's awake and starts moving around, in what is becoming more of a confined space, you'll know all about it. At times some kicks will be literally breathtaking. Your baby is also limbering up for life after delivery by learning how to suck its thumb and cry.

The bones are now fully developed but they will stay soft until after delivery. In the skull this is particularly important as it helps the baby squeeze through the birth canal. Around this time it also loses all of its downy hair (lanugo) over its skin, which is replaced by a creamy protective coating called vernix.

During these final weeks the placenta works hard allowing your antibodies to pass into your baby. This provides protection against infections that you are immune to for the first sixth months of its life, until its own immune system is mature enough to take over. This protection can be enhanced if you breastfeed, as your milk is also dripping with antibodies that your baby can absorb.

By 36 to 37 weeks your baby will be well and truly ready to make its entrance into the world, although it must be remembered that some little perishers might keep their exhausted mothers waiting for another month or so by staying put until week 42.

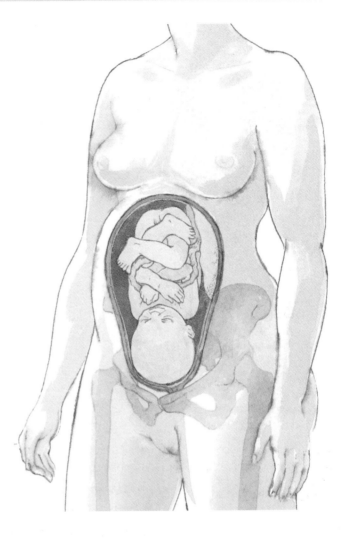

In the last month your baby's feet will be right up under your ribs and his kicks will literally take your breath away.

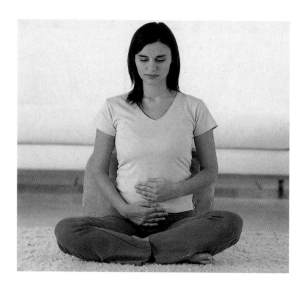

Common complaints in the third trimester

Your baby is getting bigger by the day and your body is gearing up for the big push (literally!), so inevitably there are a few more aches and pains set to try you in these last few weeks. Some are more serious than others, and most are treatable. The good news is that all these symptoms will come to an end once your baby is born.

Backache

Annoyingly, this is an inevitable consequence of pregnancy. Carrying the combined weight of your baby and your womb around in front of you will usually force you to arch your back in order to keep your centre of gravity above your feet. Obviously this position puts a strain on the muscles and joints in your back, which only gets worse as your baby gets bigger, and this causes the backache.

You can help prevent this simply by being aware of your posture and trying not to arch your back. Avoid wearing high heels and lifting heavy objects (particularly at the same time!), and always bend at the knees rather than the waist and lift using your arms and legs, rather than your back. As your pregnancy pushes on, try to put your feet up more, or at least don't stay on them too long. Finally, make sure you have a firm mattress and, if you can, get your significant other to give you a massage. After all, if he had to carry a baby he'd certainly want one!

Sciatica

The sciatic nerve is the largest and the longest nerve in the body, extending from the lower back, where it leaves the spinal cord, all the way down to the sole of the foot. There's one sciatic nerve on each side of the body but, unfortunately, in the pelvis these nerves sit right behind the enlarging womb, and when the womb hits a critical size it presses against them causing pain, tingling and numbness anywhere along their route.

While rest and warm baths can help relieve the pain of sciatica, many women suffering this condition need to be referred to a physiotherapist. Thankfully it tends to settle down just before, and certainly soon after, delivery.

Carpal tunnel syndrome

Another problem that stems from a nerve being squeezed because of pressures caused by pregnancy is carpal tunnel syndrome. In this case the culprit is the median nerve, which runs from the forearm into the wrist via a bony tunnel made up of the wrist (or carpal) bones. This tunnel contains not only this nerve but also the tendons of muscles that move the hand and fingers.

The median nerve is the one that supplies sensation to the skin of the whole of the palm of the hand (except for the little finger), along with impulses to some of the small muscles that move the fingers and thumb. In pregnancy, tissue swelling in the carpal tunnel puts pressure on the nerve and can cause a whole bunch of symptoms, ranging at its mildest from tingling and pain, to weakness of the muscles in the hand and even to a decrease in grip at the more severe end of the spectrum.

Simple actions, such as hanging the affected hand over the side of the bed, can help, but in severe cases a wrist splint may be needed or even referral to a hand specialist.

In all of these conditions simple painkillers such as paracetamol can help relieve the pain and discomfort of the symptoms, but avoid taking any anti-inflammatory drugs such as aspirin and ibuprofen, as they are not safe for use in pregnancy.

Abdominal pains

Pains in the abdomen are a common occurrence during pregnancy, as your insides get stretched in ways they've never been before, but as you reach 20 weeks and press on through the third trimester your womb will also begin tightening, which causes uncomfortable contractions known as Braxton-Hicks.

These contractions originate at the top of the womb and pass downwards, lasting between 30 and 60 seconds at a time – although occasionally they can go on for to two minutes at a time. Braxton-Hicks are often seen as practice contractions and they differ from the real thing in a number of important ways – and these differences help you to distinguish them from the genuine onset of labour. Braxton-Hicks:

- Are irregular.
- Are infrequent.
- Are non-rhythmic.
- Don't increase in frequency or intensity.

Vaginal discharge

Vaginal secretions are a part of every woman's normal life – whether pregnant or not – and when the discharge is milky white and odourless it is a sign that your body is working as it should. In pregnancy, your raised hormone levels will tend to cause you to make more of the stuff, resulting in what we medics charmingly call leucorrhoea.

For many pregnant women this will warrant the use of panty liners to keep laundry to a minimum, but avoid using tampons no matter how heavy you think it seems as this encourages infection. If your discharge becomes a bit whiffy, off-colour or it makes you itch, then you should go to see your doctor for swabs to rule out an infection.

Fluid retention and swelling

More technically called oedema, fluid retention and swelling is a normal part of pregnancy and is largely caused by the increased fluid volume that occurs. This complaint usually affects the legs, ankles and face and is often worse during hot days in the summer, when you've been on your feet for some time or if you have a lot of salt in your diet.

Your doctor needs to keep an eye out for oedema, especially if it is associated with head-aches, abdominal pains and protein in your urine (which is picked up at your antenatal checks). If this is the case then it can be a sign of a condition called pre-eclampsia (see page 113).

You can help minimize the risk and effects of oedema by:

◆ Avoiding standing for long periods.
◆ Wearing flat shoes and ditching those heels.
◆ Resting with your feet elevated on a stool rather than hanging down.
◆ Having a low-salt diet.

You can be reassured that this fluid retention and swelling tends to resolve itself after you've delivered your baby.

The later stages of pregnancy are less glamorous times, and with fluid retention and swelling of the ankles a common complaint, it's time to ditch those heels for more comfortable flatties.

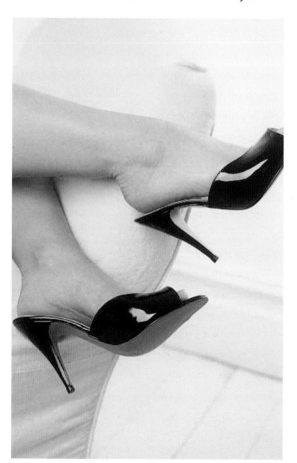

Medical problems in the third trimester

A small number of women will experience medical complications during the third trimester. All these problems wil be watched for so they can be treated quickly, but if a baby is born prematurely at this stage it will be fine.

Pre-eclampsia

The textbooks define pre-eclampsia as 'pregnancy-induced high blood pressure associated with a high level of protein in the urine', but its effects are far more wide ranging than that and it can even affect the brain, liver, kidneys, blood-clotting mechanisms and the lungs. In short, it is not good news.

Pre-eclampsia is probably the most common of the serious conditions that can occur antenatally, affecting up to 7 per cent of pregnancies and which, in its most severe form, can even be life threatening. It has been a recognized complication of pregnancy for around 150 years, but we still have no clear idea as to why it occurs.

There are, of course, many theories, and a lot of research has been carried out to try to discover which one is the most likely. A review article in the medical journal *The Lancet* (in 2005) listed four main contenders, all of which focus on problems with the formation and functioning of the placenta: in relation to the lining of its blood vessels, a conflict between the mother's and her baby's genes, an immune system abnormality or, finally, a possible problem with debris from placental cells.

Regardless of its cause, pre-eclampsia is known to be more common in first-time younger mums, older women, those expecting twins, women with diabetes and those for whom the condition runs in the family or who have had it before. Pre-eclampsia often occurs without producing any symptoms – hence the blood pressure and urine checks at antenatal appointments. But if symptoms do occur they include nausea, vomiting, ankle swelling, headaches, upper abdominal pains (because of swelling around the liver) and visual disturbances such as flashing lights.

Full-on eclampsia, for which pre-eclampsia is a warning, causes convulsions, kidney failure and coma, and can restrict the blood supply to the unborn baby. It is a very serious situation; hence the jitteriness doctors have about the condition.

Once the condition has been suspected, blood tests can determine which women need monitoring and treatment. In its most mild form this means being advised to take bed rest, regular blood pressure monitoring, blood and urine checks, and ultrasound scans of the baby to look at placental blood flow. In more severe cases medication may be needed to try to control blood pressure – although the only sure-fire way to cure the problem in this situation is to deliver the baby.

Antepartum haemorrhage

Any vaginal bleeding that occurs after 22 weeks into a pregnancy falls under this heading. Doctors will be concerned about this situation in case it is one of two potentially serious causes: placental abruption or placenta praevia.

Placental abruption occurs when part of the placenta pulls away from the wall of the uterus too early. The most likely symptoms to indicate this is happening are abdominal pain (which is sharp and sudden) and vaginal bleeding. The severity of these symptoms depends on how much of the placenta has come away.

Placental abruption can be potentially life threatening if it causes substantial blood loss, and in such cases it will result in an emergency Caesarean section or, at the very least, induction of labour (more about both of those later). However, in more minor cases doctors are most likely to adopt a wait-and-see approach which will just involve frequent ultrasound scans and close monitoring of mother and baby.

Thankfully, this is a rare problem that affects only around 1 per cent of pregnancies and is more common in women who smoke, have high blood pressure or who have had two or more babies previously.

Placenta praevia is a condition that describes what doesn't happen rather than what does. In an ideal world all placentas become attached to the upper part of the wall of the uterus – well away from the cervix – so the baby can make its exit unimpeded. In placenta praevia this doesn't happen; instead the placenta sits in the lower part of the womb either wholly or partially covering the exit. So it's right in the way. As the cervix starts to ripen and open during labour, a placenta sat in this position can become detached, which leads to painless vaginal bleeding.

This problem is often picked up at the 20-week scan when the sonographer can physically see the low-lying placenta. In many cases this will have moved by the time of a follow-up scan and will be safely out of the way of the cervix, but if it remains low then delivery by Caesarean section may well be on the

The third trimester might be a more uncomfortable time as the baby gets bigger and bigger, but it is also a period of real excitement as you get closer to meeting your baby at last.

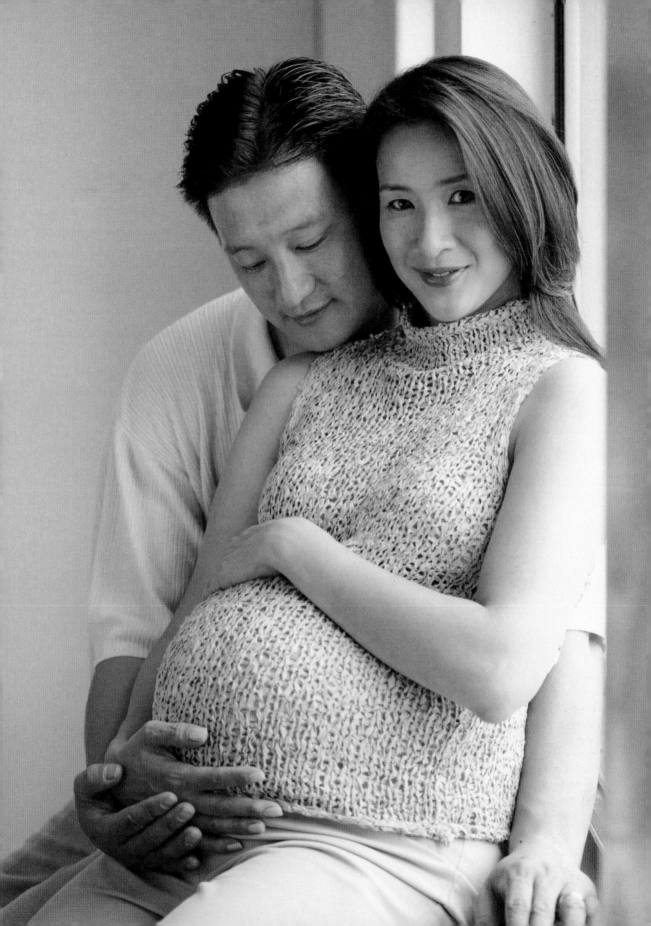

cards. If, however, events start to run away with themselves and heavy bleeding occurs before the planned delivery date, then an emergency Caesarean will be the only option.

Again, this is a rare condition that affects only 0.5 per cent of pregnancies and once more it's smokers, older mums and those who have a sizeable brood already who are most vulnerable.

Despite the fact that vaginal bleeding in later pregnancy may be a sign that you have either of these rather serious conditions, there's just as much chance that it may be down to something far more simple. Bleeding can arise from any part of your reproductive system, and polyps and erosions of the cervix are pretty common culprits.

But the bottom line is: if you experience bleeding then you need to be checked by your doctor or midwife (and probably also the maternity unit) as soon as possible. And if the smokers amongst you needed further convincing that cigarettes are bad in pregnancy, these two conditions should do the job.

Cholestasis

Now we're getting into the small print, but this condition (which affects only between 0.1 and 1 per cent of pregnant women) is still worth mentioning because it causes severe itching and jaundice in the third trimester.

Cholestasis occurs when pregnancy hormones slow down the normal flow of bile from the liver to the gallbladder. (Bile is a chemical made largely from the breakdown of old blood cells and it helps us to digest fats in our guts.) As a result, bile salts back up into the bloodstream turning the skin yellow and irritating the skin's nerve fibres, which in turn causes itching, particularly in the hands and feet. This condition will also turn your urine darker, give you paler poo and sometimes bring on nausea. It's also not great for your baby, who may become distressed and be at greater risk of premature birth.

If you develop itching your doctor or midwife can carry out a simple blood test to see if you have cholestasis but, thankfully, given how rare it is, it's unlikely to be the problem. However, if you do have the condition, treatment will focus on the relief of the itching with anti-itch and steroid creams, reducing the levels of bile acid in your blood with specific drugs and a close monitoring of your baby.

The good news is that once you've delivered your baby, the problem will quickly go away.

Antenatal depression

We've known about postnatal depression for years, but the concept of antenatal depression is a pretty recent one. It was given its highest profile in 2001 when researchers from Bristol published a paper in the *British Medical Journal* which demonstrated that as many as 10 per cent of pregnant women suffer with this condition. In fact, their study found higher depression scores for women at 32 weeks into pregnancy than eight weeks after birth – when it has been traditionally felt that the baby blues really kick in.

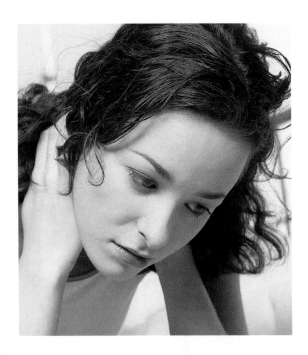

Experts now believe that there is no difference in severity of depression whether it occurs before or after giving birth, and so antenatal depression needs to be taken more seriously. (Particularly as official statistics on the causes of maternal deaths in the UK have shown that psychiatric illnesses come out on top.)

Many different things can cause antenatal depression, including hormonal changes, previous medical history of depression, being unhappy and stressed about an unplanned pregnancy, unemployment and lack of support (because a woman has no cohabiting partner or is experiencing marital disharmony). Of course, mounting life stresses – such as financial difficulties, house moves, impending wedding or divorce, or a death in the family – can also contribute.

Symptoms to look out for include:

- Low mood.
- Irritability.
- Tearfulness above and beyond the normal level in pregnancy.
- Insomnia – particularly waking early in the morning, or not getting off to sleep because your head is full of worries.
- Anxiety about situations that wouldn't normally phase you.
- Feelings of isolation and loneliness (even when you are amongst friends).
- Lack of interest in anything you normally enjoy, and also in yourself and/or your appearance.
- Loss of appetite or overeating (often called comfort eating but here taken to excess).
- Tiredness, despite rest.

New research has revealed that baby blues can kick in before the baby arrives. If you think you are suffering from antenatal depression, you should contact your doctor.

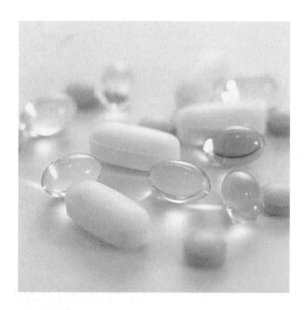

If you feel all or any of the above apply to you, then you should seek advice from your doctor or midwife because there is loads of help available which may nip things in the bud before they get out of hand. And, let's face it, if you are continually tired and have no desire either to look after yourself or to eat properly you will be doing your baby no favours at all.

It is also vital to remember that depression is an illness; it's not something you can simply shake yourself out of, and trying to pull yourself together just won't work. It's also important for your nearest and dearest to remember that, like any other illness, it is not something that you've wished on yourself and it is certainly not something you are making up to get attention. You need to get help – and the sooner the better.

Medication can be prescribed for expectant mothers for a variety of illnesses, including depression. But always consult a doctor to determine which pills are safe for your baby.

This help should include support groups and counselling, and in severe circumstances medication may need to be prescribed. Obviously this is only given when it is really needed, but if it is recommended then it is because it is considered vital to safeguard both your health and that of your baby. Aside from professional help, it's also important not to forget that talking to friends and family about how you're feeling, rather than bottling it up, can be a great, informal means of support.

Premature birth

Any child born before 37 weeks is technically considered a premature baby, with 23 weeks usually being the earliest that premature birth is ever said to occur. Premature labour happens in up to 15 per cent of all deliveries and for a variety of different reasons, including early rupture of membranes, multiple pregnancy, high blood pressure, incompetent cervix, antepartum haemorrhage and an abnormally shaped uterus. Premature birth is also brought on if the mother has a severe infection such as pneumonia or pyelonephritis (kidney infection), or because of illicit drug abuse (an estimated 25 per cent of women who use street drugs go through premature labour).

The symptoms are the same as for full-term labour, namely:

◉ Abdominal cramps.
◉ Worsening pain in the lower back.

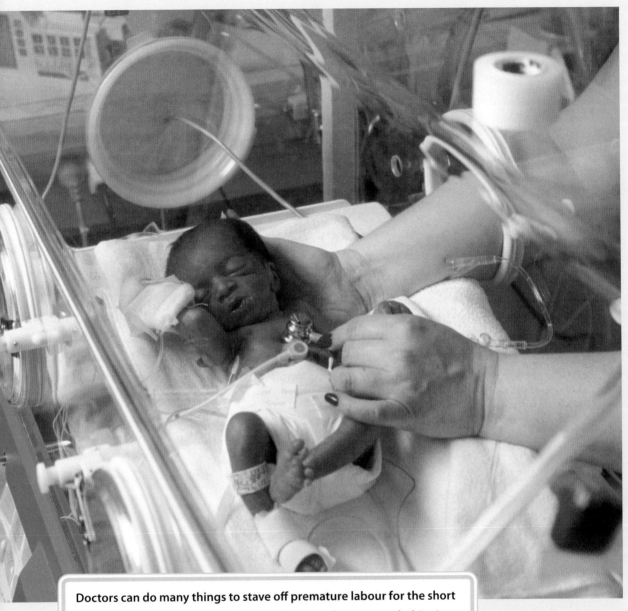

Doctors can do many things to stave off premature labour for the short term, but the biggest success story in the care of premature babies is the neonatal intensive care unit.

The technology and specialist training of the staff in these units has meant that babies born as early as 28 weeks now have an amazing 80 per cent chance of survival, while a survival rate of 100 per cent can be expected for babies born at 32 weeks.

Premature babies now have a far better chance of survival, thanks to breakthroughs in medical research and training.

- Feeling of pressure in the pelvis.
- Pink mucus discharge called a 'show'. (More of which in the next chapter.)
- Fluid gushing or trickling from the vagina as your waters break.

With enough warning there's a chance that obstetricians can slow this process down for 24 to 48 hours so that they can give the mother steroid drugs to help improve the baby's lung development. The most common drugs used for this are called tocolytics, which work by decreasing muscle contractions in the womb. In the case of women with an incompetent cervix, sutures (stitches) are often used to help keep it closed until the baby reaches a safe time for delivery.

Weakening of your pelvic floor

Your midwife is likely to bang on about the importance of performing your pelvic floor exercises throughout much of your pregnancy in order to strengthen it. Having witnessed the casualties who've failed to heed this advice, I want to echo her words – you need to give your pelvic floor a regular workout!

In some cultures, because the muscles that make up the pelvic floor tighten the vagina, women exercise them on a frequent basis in order to please their sexual partners. Other women in the less salubrious parts of Bangkok use the strength of the pelvic floor to do strange things with ping-pong balls – and I don't mean playing table tennis. In this country, though, there's a lot of ignorance about this part of our anatomy which can lead to significant problems when it comes to childbirth.

The floor in question is made up of a number of different muscles that form a hammock. This hammock sits underneath the organs in your pelvis – your bladder, intestines and, if you're a woman, uterus – and provides support for them, so that they stay where they're supposed to. It also strengthens the urinary and anal sphincters, which helps to maintain continence. In other words, the pelvic floor stops you having a wee or a poo when you don't want to.

Having a baby pushes this structure to its limits and beyond. In your pre-pregnant state the pelvic floor fits snugly around the vagina, urethra and anus, but push an 8lb baby through it and it stretches (to put it mildly) and in many cases it just doesn't want to spring back. As a result, around 30 per cent of women will have urinary incontinence after having a baby and won't dare cough or laugh for fear of leaking. A smaller, but still significant, number of women (studies estimate around 3 per cent) will lose control over faeces and around 25 per cent will not be able to hold on to their farts. And finally there

PELVIC FLOOR EXERCISES IN A NUTSHELL

The beauty of these is that, unlike other exercise regimes, they are simple to perform and don't involve you forking out to join a gym, buy an exercise bike or clad yourself from head to foot in Lycra (unless you really want to). You can do these when you're standing, sitting or lying down and anywhere you like – on the bus, in front of the tv and even while chatting on the phone. So there really is no excuse for not having a go.

◦ To find the muscles in question just stop yourself from weeing mid-stream when you're on the toilet. It's your pelvic floor muscles that allow you to do this. Next, replicate this movement when you're not on the loo. If you want to confirm you're doing this right the first time, put two fingers into your vagina when doing this exercise and you should feel a gentle squeeze. You will also feel your anus tightening at the same time and the skin between your anus and vagina (called the perineum) should move up and in.

◦ While you're doing this you shouldn't feel contractions in your thigh or abdominal muscles or your buttocks. If you do, you're doing it wrong and won't be working the correct muscles.

◦ You don't need to squeeze your legs together and you certainly don't need to hold your breath.

◦ Once you've mastered the basics you need to do frequent repetitions of the exercise in the same way you would do sit-ups to firm up your belly.

◦ It's a good idea to do a mixture of fast and slow contractions to help work the different muscles that make up the pelvic floor. For slow contractions, tighten the muscles and hold for around four seconds before releasing. Do this ten times with a gap of a further four seconds between each one. As you gain in confidence you could aim to tighten the muscles for up to ten seconds at a time. For fast contractions, only tighten the muscles for one ▶

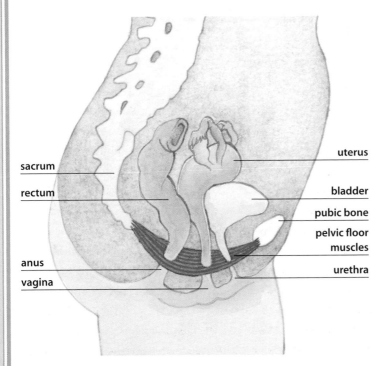

sacrum

rectum

anus

vagina

uterus

bladder

pubic bone

pelvic floor muscles

urethra

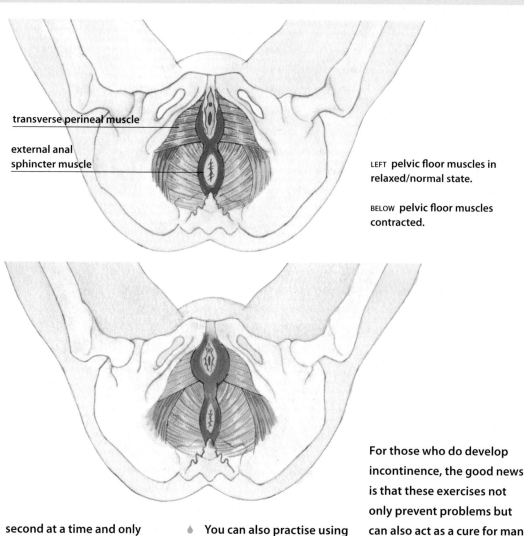

transverse perineal muscle

external anal
sphincter muscle

LEFT pelvic floor muscles in relaxed/normal state.

BELOW pelvic floor muscles contracted.

second at a time and only rest for a couple of seconds in between. Again, you should repeat this process ten times.

- The Chartered Society of Physiotherapists recommends that you repeat each of these sets of contractions around four times per day for them to be effective.

- You can also practise using these exercises as you stand, cough or sneeze.
- Keep at it and make it a regular part of your routine for the rest of your life.

Remember, if you look after your pelvic floor, it will look after you!

For those who do develop incontinence, the good news is that these exercises not only prevent problems but can also act as a cure for many women. The key is to do them regularly, but you also have to be patient, as it can take up to three months to see any benefit. If you're bothered by postnatal incontinence it's always worth a trip to see your doctor who can give further advice.

will be those who develop prolapsing of their pelvic organs, which gets worse after the menopause when the tissues become slacker still. This condition will present itself in the form of bulges in the wall of the vagina, because either the bladder or bowel – or even the uterus itself – has dropped.

All of these problems are embarrassing and debilitating, but they can easily be prevented simply by doing pelvic floor exercises. A number of studies have shown that women who do these exercises regularly have less chance of developing incontinence after giving birth and, in 2004, researchers in Norway also found that a strong pelvic floor can actually make the process of delivering your baby easier and quicker, needing less time for pushing – which can't be a bad thing.

Buying baby equipment

According to the number crunchers at Liverpool Victoria Insurance Company, the current cost of bringing up a child to the age of 21 is over £180,000 and rising. And a decent proportion of that goes on the initial running costs of a newborn baby.

Babies need to be clothed, fed, washed, changed, winded and have somewhere to lay their weary little heads at the end of a busy day; and the equipment required to fulfil all these roles doesn't come cheap.

Of course, you can start saving immediately by not following the lead of the *Hello!* magazine set by spending a fortune on designer babygros. Let's face it, if you've ever caught so much as a glimpse of a baby in action you'll know that half of what they ingest comes straight back up again and that their nappies have a horrible habit of leaking. So in less time than it takes you to dress them they're likely to have covered themselves in such a colourful array of bodily fluids that they need changing again. Designer garments are therefore completely wasted on such fashion philistines who would be just as happy in supermarket, good-value outfits or someone else's cast-offs.

You can cut the cost of these initial outgoings even further by getting a friend to hold the American tradition of a baby shower in your honour shortly before your due date. This occasion will allow friends and family to spend some of this money for you and stock you up before the big day. But whatever you choose to do, junior will have quite some shopping list. Here's a run down to get you started.

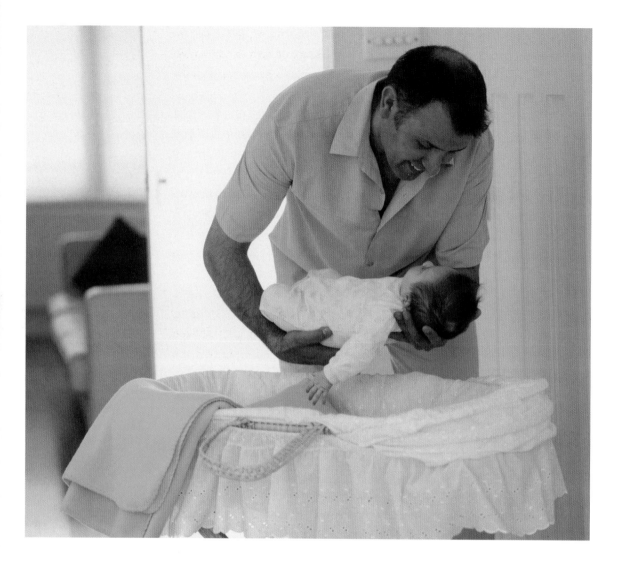

The nursery

This is a biggie. Whether your baby sleeps in your room or in its own room, you will need:

◌ A cot and/or Moses basket (for the first few weeks). You may also want to look into buying a portable travel cot, as this allows you to cart your little one around easily and, as we did, still go to friends for dinner while your baby sleeps – well, like a baby – upstairs. Baskets also have this advantage but your baby will have graduated to a full-sized cot by around four months and they are not so mobile!

◌ A mattress for the cot. This should always be new – a hand-me-down is not

As cute as your cot looks, your newborn baby will be too small to appreciate it initially, so a crib or a Moses basket is a good idea for the first few weeks.

a good idea as a bumpy mattress won't support the baby properly. There are a variety of different mattresses available, namely foam, natural fibre, hypo-allergenic and good old-fashioned spring mattresses. All are covered with PVC to help keep them clean. It doesn't matter which type you buy as long as it's firm, not soft, and it fits snugly inside the cot.

 ⬦ Blankets and sheets, but no pillows or duvets; these are not safe until your baby is one year old.

Alongside these basics there are a number of other gadgets and pieces of equipment you might want to consider:

 ⬦ Night-lights. Dim lights that plug into sockets will enable you to see what your baby's up to in the night and helps you to see what you're doing when feeding them in the wee small hours.

 ⬦ Monitors. These consist of a transmitter which sits in the nursery (or wherever else your baby is) and a receiver which you can have with you up to around 200 metres away to allow you to listen in on your baby. However, if you live in a small house or flat you will not be left in any doubt that your baby is crying – with or without the use of electrical gadgets!

 ⬦ Mobiles. These can help to soothe your baby to sleep, but you should remove them when your child can pull itself up to avoid your baby becoming tangled in them. By then you'll be sick of the tune anyway.

Clothing

Clothes don't stay clean for long, so you need a fair few if you don't want to spend your life feeding the washing machine. However, little babies quickly grow into bigger babies, so you will also need some larger-sized items in your baby's wardrobe early on to cover the eventuality that either he will take you by surprise one morning when you find his usual clothes no longer fit, or in case you produce a whopper in the first place. (It is advisable to wash all clothes and towels for your baby in non-biological washing powder before you use them to remove the manufacturer's dressing.) You will need:

 ⬦ Vests with wide necks (babies often put up a struggle when you try to dress them, so make life easy for yourself). Half a dozen or so should do.

 ⬦ Babygros. Again, 6–10 should be enough.

 ⬦ Four to five sleepsuits for bedtime.

 ⬦ Cotton socks to do the job of shoes for the first couple of months.

 ⬦ Muslin squares. We came to these pretty late in our house and only had them with our third baby. They're a great form of over the shoulder protection for parents, as they soak up possets and dribble and the follow through most babies produce from their mouths after you've given them a pat to wind them. It certainly saves on embarrassing stains on your best clothes.

◊ If it's winter, then stock up on hats, gloves and an all-in-one suit or coat. For summer babies, vests alone may well do.

Bathtime

You can wash your baby in your own bath tub as long as there's only a shallow water level. There are also a wide range of bath supports available, which make bathtime a safe procedure by supporting the baby for you so that you have a free hand. When they're very little, the sink might even suffice – just be careful of the taps. Plastic baby baths, however, are quite cheap so you may want to invest in one of these.

You'll also need:

◊ Cotton wool balls – which let you get water into delicate little places.

◊ Baby bath oil, although if your baby has eczema this will need to be stopped as it dries their skin out.

◊ Towels. There are some lovely ones available that have hoods which help keep your baby warm while you dry them.

Changing equipment

Let's face it, changing nappies in the first few weeks seems a never-ending job and you will marvel at how much time you spend doing it. Even as they get older, nappy changing is a regular chore in the baby's day, so it's worth making it as pleasurable, or at least as hassle-free, a procedure as it can be!

A wipeable mat or two will certainly come in handy, as these can easily be disinfected when your little one escapes from your grasp while you're cleaning them and spreads their bodily effluent all over it – and most likely you as well!

You can also buy smart changing tables, which allow you to keep all your kit inside them and also provide a platform at an ergonomic height for you to carry out these procedures without hurting your back.

And, of course, you need nappies. Loads and loads of them. You can either choose disposables, which will clog up landfill sites for centuries but are convenient to use (although eco-friendly disposables are now available – at a price), or opt for cloth nappies which either you or one of a burgeoning number of laundry services can wash and re-use.

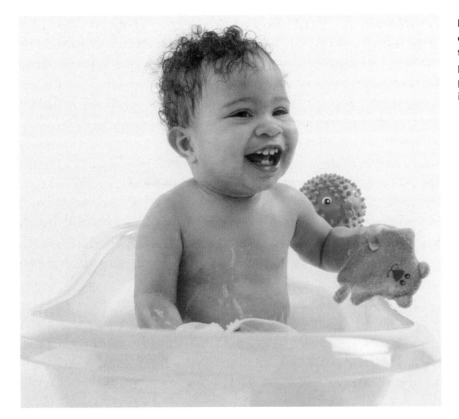

Plastic baby baths are cheap, safe and hygienic to use, and perfect for parents nervous of putting a newborn into a great big bath.

Transport

As with all the gear I've already mentioned, it is vital that all baby-transport equipment conforms to British and European safety standards, so always check the label before you buy. You should never buy a second-hand car seat if it looks damaged or you suspect or know that it has been in an accident.

Car seats

It's now a legal requirement for children to be seated in one sort of car seat or other until the age of 11, and anyone who even considers carrying a baby in their arms on a car journey needs their head tested (not to mention their suitability for parenting). Many hospitals will even prevent you taking a baby home in a car without a seat. Car seats come in varying sizes depending on the age and weight of your child – with the seats for new babies being smaller and rear-facing. These can be strapped into either the front or back seats of the car, but if you have air bags fitted you must have them deactivated as they are not safe for use with child car seats.

Pushchairs

There's a great deal of choice when it comes to these and many parents-to-be will have a preconceived idea about what shape their baby's wheels should take. When selecting your ride of choice, remember that you will have to get it in and out of the car or bus, through the crowds in shopping malls, down slopes in the park and often up and down steps. So go for one that's light, manoeuvrable, easy to fold up and, crucially, will fit into your boot if you have a car. Do explain to other carers of your baby how the buggy works – my parents once got completely stuck and ended up driving home with the pushchair still erected because I hadn't explained how it worked!

For newborns, your pushchair should allow them to lie flat and be able to face either direction. It also needs to be comfortable for you, so adjustable handles are a must, as is a three-point harness – so that your baby doesn't fly out as you bounce it downstairs – and plenty of room to store your shopping bags to make pushing the pram easier when laden with groceries.

Some people choose a pushchair because of its looks, others for its practicality. Whatever you choose, make sure it does what you want it to do.

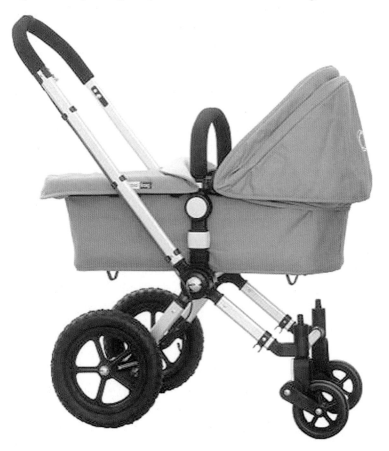

Of course, for the fitness fanatics and outward bounders amongst you there are all-terrain three-wheelers available so you can take your baby jogging with you, but for most parents the bog standard varieties will be just the job.

Feeding

The choice for new mothers is whether to breast or bottle feed – and that's something your midwife will chat to you about (and that I will discuss further in Chapter 6).

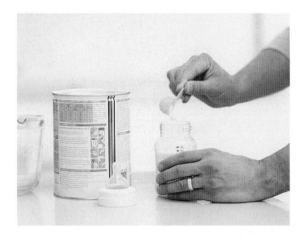

Formula milk has come on in leaps and bounds in recent years and now a variety of brands are available for all different stages of your baby's development.

Breastfeeding

If you decide to breastfeed then you'll need to buy some nursing bras so that you can pop your boobs out easily when and wherever they are called upon to come up with the goods. It's also worth buying some breast pads to mop up any extraneous production before it soaks through your clothes.

A breast pump is always a good idea so that you can express and store your milk. Doing this enables someone else to feed your baby with a bottle when you're not around or when you fancy a sleep or some time out. They are also a godsend if you need to relieve the pressure on your breasts when they are literally full to bursting. These pumps are either electrical or manual, but the automatic variety comes out on top where ease and convenience is concerned.

If you're going to express milk then you'll also need some bottles, teats, cleaning and sterilizing equipment, and you can also buy bags in which to freeze milk for future use.

Bottle feeding

Again, you will need bottles, sterilizers and other cleaning equipment and you'll also need some powdered milk (or formula) which your midwife will advise you about after delivery.

Birthplan

So you're almost there after months of hard work. You've had to ride the waves of nausea, you need a search party to find your feet and you couldn't get comfortable in a room full of nothing but cushions and fluffy things with a personal slave to tend to your every whim. But, and here's the good news, there's now

Birthplan

Name: Sarah Peel
Birth attendant: Colin Peel

Labour:
I would consider a sweep if I go over my due date, but I would prefer not to be induced if at all possible.
I would like to be walking around and have minimal monitoring once labour has started. If a birthing pool is available I would like to spend the labour in it, but not necessarily give birth in it.
I would like to bring in some music for the labour period.

Pain relief:
I would like to use gas and air and would consider an epidural if the pain gets too uncomfortable. I do not want to use pethidine.

Position for birth:
Have no preference for position for birth.

Cutting the cord:
My partner does not wish to do this.

The birth
I would like my partner and the midwife present but would prefer not to have anyone else there unless it is essential.
I would like to avoid unnecessary medical intervention if possible, especially a Caesarean. I am happy for my partner to make these decisions for me if I am unable to.
I am happy to be given the injection to speed up the delivery of the placenta.

Breastfeeding:
I would like to breastfeed and would like the baby given to me after birth to try to get feeding going. I would like the baby cleaned first, though.

Vitamin K:
I am happy for the baby to be given a vitamin K injection.

a light at the end of the tunnel and the only thing left between you and your baby is a few hours of labour and the odd twinge of pain or two…

So now you get the chance to choose how you would like this baby of yours to come into the world; you can get your wishes down onto paper in a birth-plan. Of course, this isn't legal and binding, and Nature may well rip it up on the big day and take its own route, but it's a way of letting those who are going to look after you through labour know how you'd like things to go if circumstances allow.

The plan should cover such things as:

- Where you want to have your baby: either at home or in hospital, on dry land or under water.
- Whether you want to play your George Michael CD to soothe you through labour or listen to a bit of Nirvana while you're pushing.
- Who's going to be there supporting you through the whole business.
- Whether you want to be induced if things drag on.
- How much prodding and poking you want from clinical staff to assess progress.
- The types of pain relief you'd be happy with/desperate for!
- Your chosen position (which should be comfortable, but not bizarre).
- Your thoughts about Caesareans and assisted delivery (ventouse and forceps).
- Whether you want to allow your placenta to be left to be delivered naturally or whether you want an injection to get it out as soon as possible.
- Whether your partner would like to cut the cord.
- Whether you are happy for the vitamin K jab to be administered to your baby (see page 182).

Of course, the minute things kick off and your labour gets into full swing, your ideas might change, but if you've at least considered your options you won't feel out of your depth once the big moment arrives. And it's coming soon.

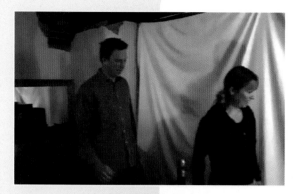

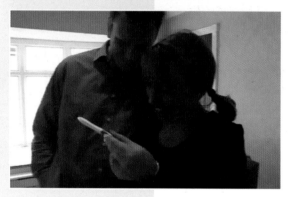

Jane and Simon discovered they were having a third baby just as they were about to experience another major upheaval – moving and renovating a new house. Not surprisingly, this triggered stress for Jane, who then developed antenatal depression.

Antenatal depression

When psychologists produce lists of which stressful life events can have an impact on our mental health, pregnancy always scores pretty highly – along with the death of a loved one, divorce, moving house and Christmas! Most of us can cope with dealing with any of these situations if they come along one at a time, but if they gang up and two or three happen at the same time, then it can spell trouble.

For Jane and Simon the first of these common stressful life events was pregnancy, but this was coupled with the stress of moving house, which they cranked up a gear by deciding to completely renovate their new home as well. This meant that they had to move into temporary accommodation so that the building work could be completed while Jane was still pregnant.

This couple already had two daughters, one aged four and the other five. They had successfully conceived both by having sex on days thirteen and fourteen of Jane's cycle, so they decided to follow this plan in order to conceive their third child.

Despite this low frequency of sex, Jane became pregnant quite quickly, in January 2006. They learned of this new addition to the family not long before they had to depart their home, so Jane's tears of joy at a positive pregnancy test were tinged with some of trepidation about how she would cope with all the building work going on in the background.

As a result, Jane didn't cope well and found the upheaval particularly stressful. Soon the renovations became a real bone of contention between the couple as the job seemed to be taking forever, even though, as a builder, Simon was directing the work himself.

Thankfully the pregnancy itself progressed really well, with a low risk result for the triple blood test and a happily normal 20-week ultrasound scan. But as time went on the stress of the work on the house really began to get to Jane, compounded by the fact that Simon didn't share her anxiety

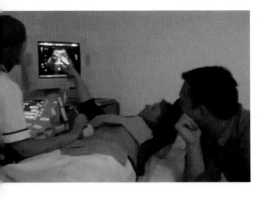

and was viewing the whole process quite calmly.

Towards the end of the pregnancy Jane and Simon finally moved into their new house – which was absolutely stunning. However, Jane was faced not with the simple job of getting on with 'nesting' ready for the arrival of their baby, but a massive clear up operation in order to simply make their house a home in time for the baby making its entrance.

Not surprisingly when experiencing all this stress, Jane became very low and tearful – on one occasion she even felt so bad that she thought about how it would be easy to crash her car into a wall and not be around any more.

At an antenatal appointment with her midwife soon after, Jane became very emotional and told her how she had been feeling. She was shocked when she was told that she was suffering with antenatal depression. Like many women, Jane didn't know that such a condition existed, let alone how common it is, and so she was enormously relieved to find that she wasn't just going mad and that there was even help available.

Still, it took Jane a while until her mood picked up, particularly as Simon felt completely unable to comprehend why she was feeling the way she was. After all, with a new house and a new baby on the way, the last thing he felt she should be was depressed. But after a month or so Jane did begin to feel better and happier, and in October 2006 she was delighted to give birth to her longed-for third child, Ruby.

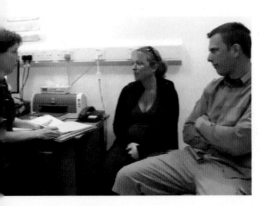

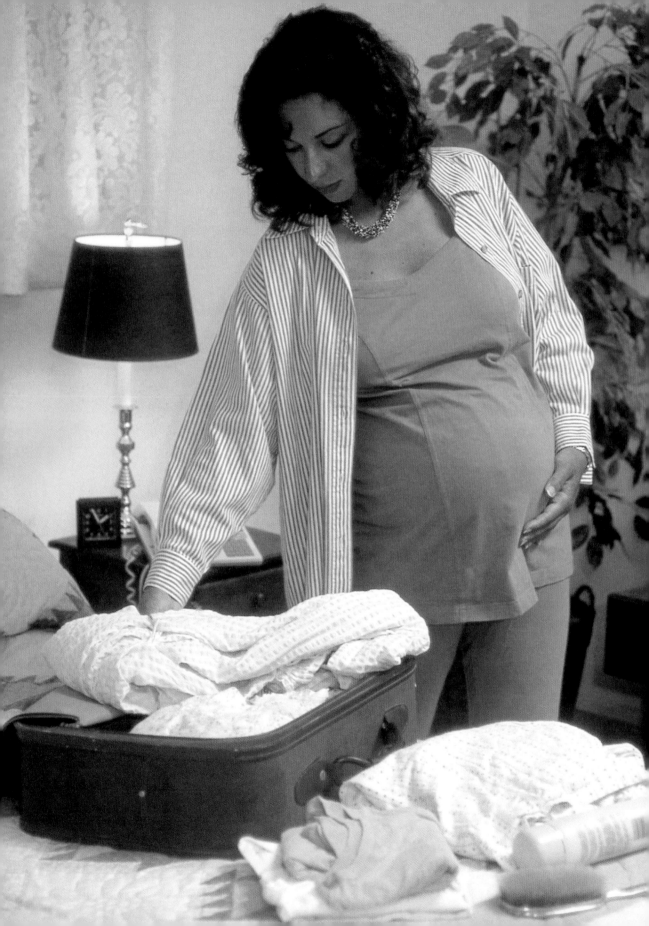

chapter 5

Prepare for D-day

Robert Baden-Powell (the founder of the boy scouts movement and a man not often quoted in books about pregnancy) has instilled a motto in generations of young protégés: be prepared. This is as vital as you head towards childbirth as it is for any group of spotty youths embarking on a camping trip.

Of course, on one level there's no excuse for not being ready the minute labour begins, as you've had a whopping nine months' warning that this event is going to happen. However, it must be remembered that although you've known your expected date of delivery all that time, it's only a rough estimation, not an immutable date like Christmas Day or Boxing Day – which, of course, always fall exactly on the dates they're supposed to.

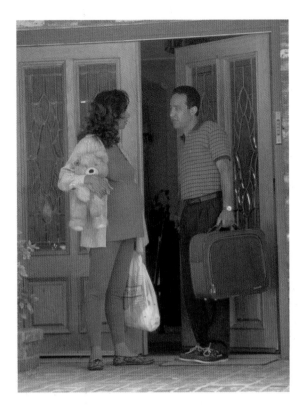

Have your case packed and waiting in a convenient spot in the house, so when Nature calls, you're ready for the off.

So don't leave it to the last minute to sort out your final preparations because you never know when that last minute may be – and here I speak from personal experience. We have three children and none of them arrived straightforwardly. Our first, who was born three weeks early, made his entrance the night we'd been out celebrating our wedding anniversary. With a pregnant wife as ready-made chauffeur, I'd been able to enjoy a few celebratory drops of ale and drunkenly slipped into bed just after midnight. Just two hours later I was woken by a sharp nudge in the back accompanied by the rather shocking announcement that my wife had just felt (and heard) a pop in her nether regions and that she was now busy wetting the bed.

Given my earlier alcohol consumption it took rather longer than it should have done for my medical mind to register the fact that my wife hadn't suddenly become incontinent, but that her waters had broken and our little boy was on his way. We rang the midwife who told us to go in to the hospital. So, with me still over the limit, my poor wife had to drive us both to hospital while her nethers leaked amniotic fluid and her womb started to contract alarmingly.

In the end, we made it to hospital with plenty of time to spare as her contractions seemed to stop the minute we passed through the maternity unit's doors. And it was another seven hours, after my hangover had well and truly kicked in, before we had our first glimpse of our newborn baby.

Our second son was a bit better behaved and at least waited until 38 weeks to make his presence felt. Unfortunately I was working on the paediatric wards when my wife's waters went, but luckily in the same hospital where she was due to give birth. Fortunately her parents had arrived for Easter so her dad was able to take her in (something which confused the receptionist on the labour ward no end, as she seemed convinced he must be the baby's father!).

Despite being rushed off our feet, my consultant very kindly let me join them so I could see little Sam being born, while all paediatric admissions were re-routed to another hospital in the city (which went down well with my colleagues there!). They also let me stay with my wife and son on the postnatal

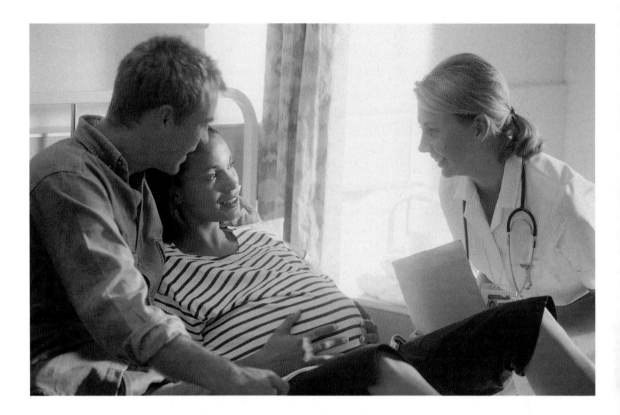

ward for an hour or so before calling me back to my own ward so I could make up for lost time and work through the rest of the night.

And finally, there was our third son, who decided to come at four o'clock in the morning, some four weeks early, while we were away on holiday in Devon! We were staying in a cottage in a rocky bay down by the sea. There was no land line and no mobile phone signal, and knowing that the local cottage hospital would be closed at that ungodly hour, I had visions of us having to call in the local vet to do the honours.

Thankfully we managed to get through to the hospital in Barnstaple, some 20 miles away, and so we sped off, zigzagging along tortuous country lanes while trying to avoid the kamikaze wildlife which leapt at us from the hedge-rows (there were no casualties!) as my wife's contractions became closer and ever more extreme.

When we eventually arrived we were relieved to find that, in the rather sleepy countryside, there was an excellent maternity unit, and after two hours of sweat and toil (and just a little effort on the part of my wife) we were a family of five.

When you arrive at the hospital you will be assessed by a midwife and either asked to stay or told to go home until the labour really gets going.

Thankfully it all worked out in the end, but none of these scenarios featured anywhere in the birthplans we'd prepared.

Oh, and there's no need to feel smug if you're planning a home delivery either – you can be caught on the hop too, as a friend of ours, and ex-midwife to boot, will testify. Her third child was so quick out of the starting blocks that she nearly experienced a water birth down the U-bend of the toilet.

So, the take-home message really is: be prepared.

Getting ready

Being prepared for birth is not just about breathing, birthplans and having the car full of petrol (but these are all very important aspects of getting ready for the off). It's also a good idea to have a bag packed at least four weeks before your due date ready for your trip to hospital.

Your hospital bag

Don't leave it until you can't speak through contractions to get this lot together. If you are going any distance from your home, it's also sensible to pack your bag in the car with you in case you get caught out.

Your antenatal class will probably give you a list of things to pack, but if not, a few essentials include:

◊ Something to wear in labour, such as an old cotton nightie or baggy T-shirt. You need to be comfortable while allowing easy access for the midwife to your delicate little places and eventually your exiting baby. Bear in mind that whatever you wear is likely to collect some interesting stains, so don't pack your best silky number.

◊ Plenty of pairs of knickers – again, these may be rendered beyond the help of even the strongest washing powder, so don't take your favourites.

◊ Maternity pads (they're like industrial-strength sanitary towels and as thick as a 13-tog duvet), because you will leak a bit for a good few days afterwards.

◊ Wash kit, toothbrush and paste, make-up and, obviously, a hairbrush.

◊ Clean nighties and going-home clothes for you for when it's all over. (Don't pack your favourite skinny jeans – you won't fit into those again for a good few months, so bring outsize clothes or maternity outfits instead.)

◊ Nursing bras and breast pads if you are hoping to breastfeed.

◊ Clothes, nappies and a blanket for when the baby gets its first taste of the outdoors. (Pack according to the season, but bear in mind babies feel the cold and a blanket is still a good idea on a warm summer evening as you go home.)

- Some snacks and glossy mags to keep you going and any music you want played if your hospital has a CD or cassette player.
- Your maternity record book.
- A present for any other children 'from the baby'.
- A mobile phone or some change so your partner can ring round the news.
- The baby's car seat.
- A map – if, like us, you're not at home and need to find the nearest maternity hospital! (This one's obviously optional.)

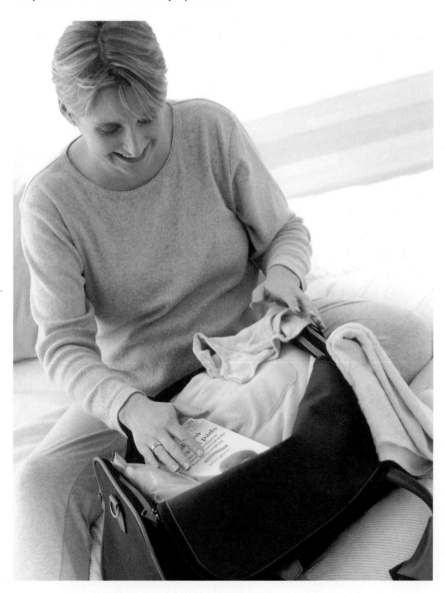

Pack a few essentials for labour, but remember that your partner might be in and out of hospital to see you, so you don't need everything but the kitchen sink!

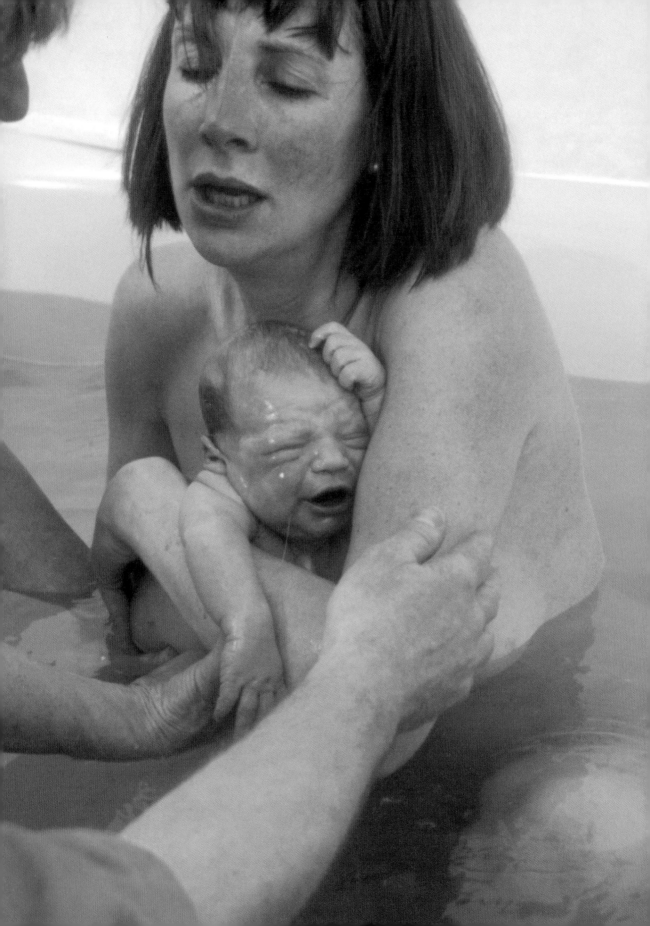

Equipment for home delivery

Having a baby at home may seem less hassle because, in theory, you should have everything you need with you, but a little advance preparation will prevent your partner turning the house upside down to find the towel and nightie you wanted to use during labour. Laying the right groundwork – literally – will also reduce the amount of clearing up you'll have to do once you are holding your newborn in your arms.

So, dig out and put to one side (in an obvious place) the following:

- Plastic sheet to protect the bed, carpet or sofa.
- Old sheets – in case bodily fluids miss the above protection.
- Snacks and drinks.
- Cotton wool and tissues.
- Bin liners.
- A basin for water.
- Something to wrap your baby in immediately after it's born, like an old towel.
- The same old nighties and knickers as above.
- The same industrial sanitary towels as above.

Other considerations

If you have other children they'll need someone to look after them while you're giving birth, whether you're going into hospital or having a home birth, so line up someone who is willing and able to help at short notice or in the middle of the night. Then have a back-up plan in case plan A goes pear-shaped.

Make sure your partner knows where they're taking you and where they can leave the car when you get there. Most hospitals these days charge you to park in their grounds, and there's nothing like getting a parking ticket or finding a wheel clamp on your vehicle to take the shine off the joy of heading home with a new baby.

Practise fitting the car seat well before the first contractions; they can be tricky beggars to strap in at the best of times and even more so when you're under pressure and have a hungry, wailing baby in your ear.

Make sure your cupboards and your freezer are well stocked so your baby's first trip out isn't to the supermarket. That's a stress you really won't need.

If you're planning a home birth make sure you have all the kit ready. When my sister-in-law was born my wife's father only just made it back in time from the hardware store with a plastic tablecloth to put on the floor, because they were completely unprepared for what a messy business childbirth can be.

Although birthing pools are available in some maternity units, there might not be one free on the day. So if you really want a water birth, home is where you will be guaranteed the opportunity.

Getting to the big push

Going through labour and delivering a baby vaginally is one of the few experiences we humans have to remind us that we are part of the animal kingdom. As our brains have evolved, the need to travel everywhere on foot as our mammalian cousins do has been supplanted by various means of transport such as cars, planes and space shuttles. We no longer have to hunt and kill our own food, and with the advent of online shopping we don't even have to leave the house to get hold of it now. Our need for shelter has also been taken care of in ways that even our ancestors of just 100 years ago could not have dreamed of.

But, unless you're booked in for a Caesarean for some reason, in order to have a baby you have to go through the same rigmarole as lions, apes and whales and push it out of a small hole in your pelvis. And short of licking the vernix off it as they do, the smells and sensations involved in twenty-first century childbirth are the same as they've been since pre-history. This fact I'm sure contributes in some biological way to the emotions of the situation and helps us forge the natural bonds we have with our children as soon as they emerge.

The actual process of labour is clinically split into three stages, each of which will provide you with different challenges and symptoms which are the same for all natural births whether at home or in hospital. (If you have a Caesarean section, particularly if it's a planned one, then you may miss out on all three, so Caesarean births will be covered separately later.)

The whole process, from start to finish, will take a variable amount of time from woman to woman. But as a guide, the average length of labour for a first-timer is around 8–12 hours, although it can be much longer or possibly even shorter (if you're lucky!) while for a second baby (when the body knows what it's doing) it's generally only 6–8 hours. I say only, but having never been through it myself I'm sure that eight hours feels like a lifetime, so apologies.

Induction of labour

If you reach 42 weeks with no sign of normal labour kicking in, and your baby is dragging its heels, then it is most likely your midwife and/or doctor will suggest inducing labour. If your baby is coaxed into coming out at this time there's a lot of good evidence to show that this cuts down the chances of Caesarean section, instrumental delivery and, most importantly, foetal distress.

Induction might also be recommended to bring on labour in mothers who have diabetes, high blood pressure or pre-eclampsia, and where it's felt that the baby may be in trouble if you wait for labour to start naturally.

The countdown to holding your baby in your arms at long last has begun. But only Nature knows how long the wait will be.

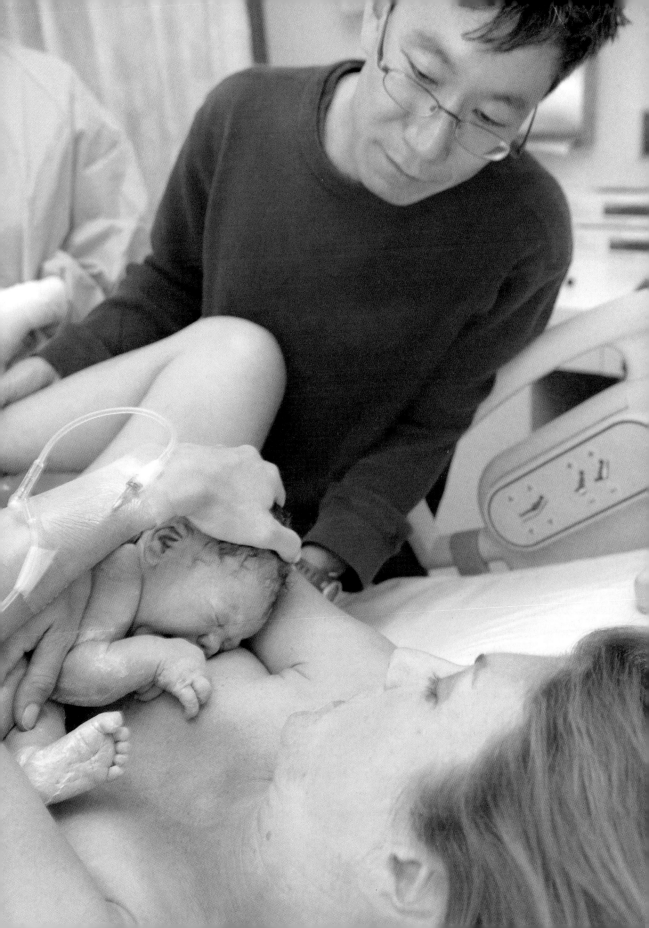

Methods used

The most simple method of induction is generally known as a 'stretch and sweep'. This involves your midwife or doctor popping a finger into your cervix and trying to separate the membranes from the cervix by making a circular sweeping motion.

This procedure is a little uncomfortable, but it may be enough to get things going without the need for any other induction methods.

The next most common method used is to try to help your cervix to ripen. Successful induction is most likely if this process has already started, and an internal examination will therefore be carried out to suss out how things are going. If success is thought to be likely, then synthetic prostaglandins (usually in the form of a pessary or gel) are used to speed up ripening of the cervix by popping a dose into your vagina.

These drugs alone may well be enough to kick-start labour, but if not then there are a couple of other methods that are commonly used:

◊ Amniotomy: this is the technical term for when a midwife breaks your waters using a plastic hook.

THE SCIENCE OF CHILDBIRTH

So your nine months are up and you're ready for the off: your bag's packed, there's petrol in the car and you've stocked up on sanitary pads. But why on earth should your baby want to be born now? Why, after all these months in a protective, warm and cosy environment, where someone else feeds and waters it, should it feel the need to leave all that luxury behind for the cold uncertainty of the outside world? And, for that matter, what makes the muscular uterus, which has happily expanded for 40 weeks, suddenly want to contract?

Well to be honest, we're not completely sure. The ancient Greeks (those in the know like Hippocrates) thought it was because the baby had reached a size where the mother could no longer feed it, so it had no choice but to jump ship. But now we know that's not true, otherwise we would see more babies being born prematurely to avoid being starved to death in the womb.

Of course, unlike our ancestors, we have the advantage of technology to carry out scientific research into the triggers of childbirth, rather than relying on observations and guesses. For ethical reasons, much of what we've discovered has come from studies on other mammals, and as a result it now seems that the main instigator of the process is not the physical size of the baby, but its hormones.

The story (so far) goes something like this:
As we saw in Chapter 1,

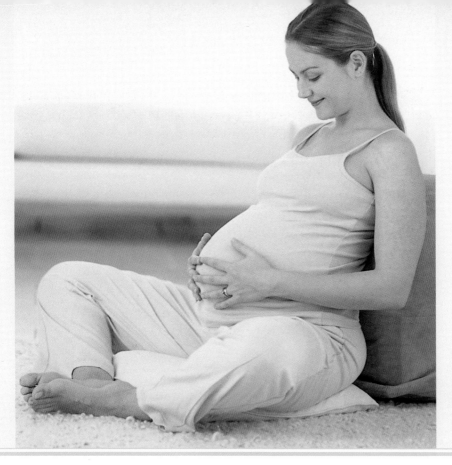

Whether you've done it before or you're a first-time mother, the last few days of having your baby in the womb are special and exciting.

from very early on in pregnancy the placenta produces a hormone called progesterone to keep the muscle fibres of the womb nice and relaxed; and this allows the uterus to expand as the baby grows.

It does this by reducing the sensitivity of the uterine muscle to the effects of another hormone, oxytocin. This hormone is also produced throughout pregnancy, but when labour begins it works to stimulate muscle contractions.

At the end of pregnancy there is a rise in the level of other hormones called cortisol and corticotrophin. Some scientists believe that this is triggered by the placenta, while others think it is due to hormone secretions from the baby's brain.

But however it happens, the end result is that these hormones stimulate a rise in the level of oestrogen and also in that of chemicals called prostaglandins.

Oestrogen has the opposite effect to progesterone and

makes the womb more sensitive to oxytocin, so it now begins to contract. Meanwhile, prostaglandins cause the cervix to begin to dilate and, Bob's your uncle, your baby's on its way.

Of course, the observant among you will note that this hasn't provided any explanation as to what might switch this hormone cascade on in the first place. However, there's a good reason for this: the scientists are still trying to fathom it out.

- Oxytocin infusion: this is a man-made version of the hormone which stimulates your womb to contract and is given through a needle in your vein as an infusion, via a pump that the midwife will use to regulate the dose.

Another method (and one best tried at home rather than on the delivery ward) is to have sex. Not only does semen contain natural prostaglandins, but having an orgasm can stimulate your own prostaglandins too. It's also got to be a lot more pleasant than having a healthcare professional fiddle about.

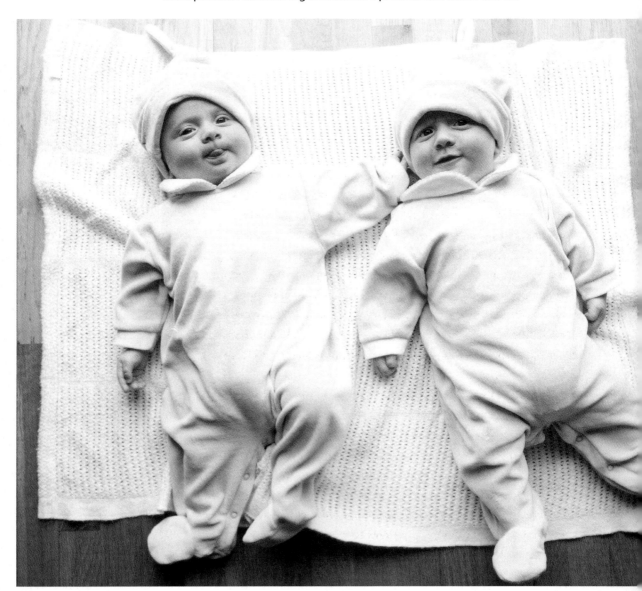

Some people also advocate acupuncture, homoeopathy, various herbal medicines and eating hot curries and fresh pineapple as methods for bringing on labour. But unfortunately there's little scientific evidence for the effectiveness of any of these theories, and a hot curry might just give you diarrhoea – and your undercarriage is going to get uncomfortable enough in the very near future as it is, so it's probably best to give that one a miss.

If all these attempts fail and labour is not induced, then the only other option available to you to get the baby out safely is to undergo a Caesarean section.

TWIN DELIVERY

Pre-term labour is much more common in twins, with almost 45 per cent of women going into labour before 37 weeks, and because of the limited space inside the womb, at least one of the twins may be breech. (It's reckoned that in around 40 per cent of cases both will be head down, whereas in a further 40 per cent one of them will be breech and in 10 per cent of cases both twins will be in the breech position.)

As with the antenatal period, twins are more likely to have problems when it comes to labour, so delivery is usually carefully planned. In fact, it is likely that labour for mothers of twins will be induced before reaching 40 weeks, and both babies will be monitored closely throughout labour. Your delivery room will be overrun with clinical staff; you will need a midwife for each baby, a senior obstetric doctor, an anaesthetist, a paediatrician and a specialist children's nurse (at the very least).

If both babies are positioned head down in the womb, then vaginal delivery can certainly be attempted as normal and it can also be tried even if one is breech. However, you can expect a rather quicker decision to proceed to Caesarean if there are problems than you would in the case of a single baby. It is therefore not unusual to have one baby born vaginally and the other by Caesarean. But this is by no means definite and many women can also find themselves pushing out twins completely naturally without any doctors interfering.

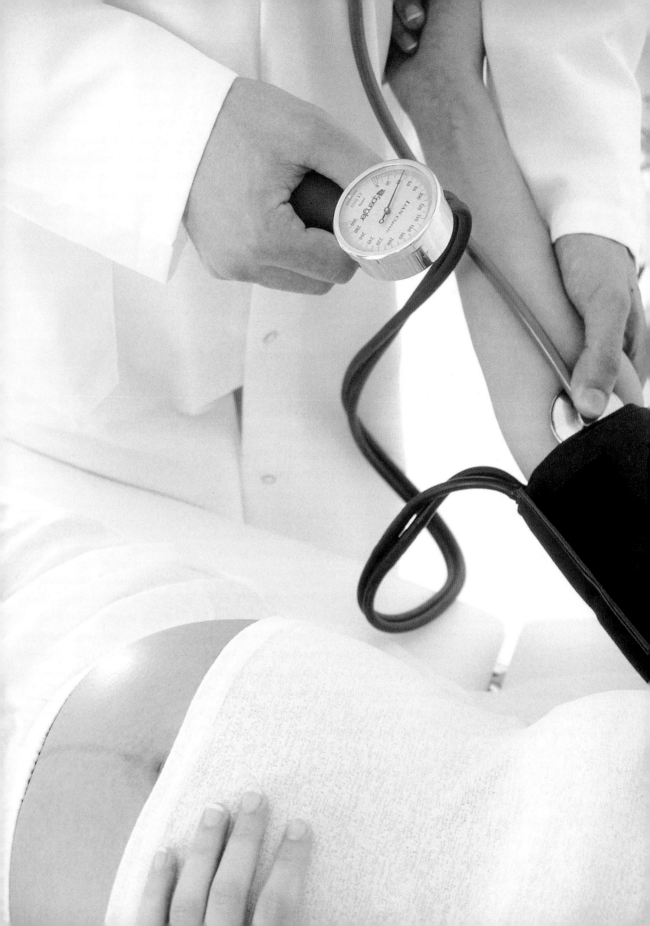

First stage labour

This stage runs from the onset of labour right up to the point when the cervix (neck of the womb) is fully dilated. It's further split into what's called the latent phase, which is the contracting bit, and the active phase, which begins at full dilatation. Of course, first you need to know whether you're really in labour or not.

Diagnosing labour

So how do you know if what you're experiencing is just the mother of all Braxton-Hicks contractions or actually the real thing? As you can imagine, it's important for you to be able to make this distinction so you know whether to grin and bear it until it settles down or frantically get your bag, get your birth partner and get in touch with your midwife.

If it is the real thing then the following will probably happen:

◦ Your womb will start contracting. Initially this discomfort will be manageable and may be helped by sitting in the bath, but as things progress these contractions will become more regular, progressively stronger, longer lasting, more frequent and, as a result, more painful.

◦ Your waters may break (in about 12 per cent of women this happens before their contractions kick in). You'll know all about this because you'll get a gush of clear fluid from your vagina and down your leg. If it's brown in colour it means the baby has had its first poo inside you and may be in distress, in which case you need to contact the midwife immediately. If the fluid is blood-stained, that could signify a haemorrhage and she needs to know about that pretty urgently too.

◦ You have a 'show'. About two-thirds of women have one of these; it is experienced as a blood-stained mucus discharge which is ejected into your pants as the mucus plug in the cervix is dislodged so your baby can make its exit.

Once you're really convinced that proper labour is underway, you need to call your midwife and tell her what's been happening so that she can either pack her bags and head round to your house (if that's where you're having it), or tell you to get yourself to hospital. Contrary to the way labour is depicted on telly, you don't immediately need to dial 999 when it all kicks off, unless your midwife advises you to.

When you arrive at hospital in labour, your midwife will run through all the procedures you'll be familiar with from antenatal appointments, including taking your blood pressure.

What happens next?

When you arrive at the hospital, or your midwife turns up at your home, you will be examined to make sure you are definitely in labour, before you start settling yourself in for the next few hours, and to make sure that that rest of your body is in good enough shape for the job in hand. So all the usual suspects will be checked:

- Temperature.
- Pulse.
- Blood pressure.
- Urine.

Your midwife will then do the first of many internal examinations and stick a couple of fingers into your vagina to see how dilated your cervix is (the labour ward is not the place to feel shy, but if this is your second baby you will have no inhibitions about this anyway).

Of course, your midwife will also check your belly to see which way round your baby is and whether or not its head is engaged. She will also have a listen to your baby's heartbeat – either with the same type of doppler machine that's been used in your antenatal checks or, more likely in hospital, with a cardiotocograph machine (CTG). [See page 157.]

If after all that it seems like you're going great guns and labour is progressing rapidly, then you may be moved into a room on the labour ward. If things have started but are on a go slow, you will pretty much be left to stew for a bit longer and advised to settle down with a good book or a Sudoku until things hot up. If nothing much is happening at all and your cervix is shut tighter than the gates of Fort Knox, you may well be sent home (or if you're at home, your midwife may leave you to carry on with her rounds of other expectant mothers and will check back with you later).

Pain relief

Of course, if you are in labour then chances are you will have been feeling the pain of your contractions for the whole time you were being prodded and poked by your midwife. So hopefully once she's done her bit, rather than popping to the canteen for her coffee break, she will sort you out with some pain relief. You may well have set out clearly in your birthplan the types of analgesia you do and don't want, but if you've decided to wing it instead and are making it up as you go along, here are the options.

None at all

Not many women opt for the grin-and-bear it approach but it is mandatory for the followers of some religions such as Scientology, who are also supposed to stay silent throughout the process. Ouch!

'Natural' approaches

Those who prefer not to use drugs for pain relief in childbirth can often be helped by alternative treatments such as acupuncture, reflexology, massage, homeopathy, hypnosis and aromatherapy. While there's not a lot of scientific evidence to prove these methods actually curb the pain, except in the case of acupuncture, they certainly seem to help women to manage it better.

Transcutaneous electrical nerve stimulation (TENS)

This is a more technical version of rubbing yourself when you've been hurt in order to ease the pain. The machine delivers a low-level electrical current to the skin which blocks pain signals from the uterus. It's completely safe throughout labour and is at its most effective during the early stages, but might also work sufficiently to postpone the need for stronger pain relief later on.

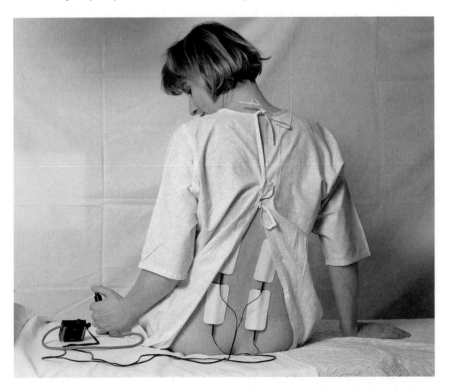

TENS machines are effective at easing the pain of labour; however, bear in mind that they do restrict movement and cannot be used in a birthing pool or the bath.

THE LOW-DOWN ON EPIDURALS

After numbing a patch on your skin on your back, the anaesthetist will pop a fine needle between two of the vertebrae in your lower back. Through this they will thread some plastic tubing (catheter) until it arrives in the fat of your epidural space (the space between the bone of your spinal column and the dura, which is the fibrous tissue covering your spinal cord and brain).

Salt solution is injected first to make sure the tubing is in the right place, and then a local anaesthetic follows to complete the process.

This procedure takes around a quarter of an hour and, once the anaesthetic is squirted in, it will take just a few minutes for your lower abdomen and pelvis to feel completely numb. Your legs won't be affected as they would have been in the old days, so you don't need to worry that you will be paralyzed during labour.

Once the catheter is in place, your level of anaesthesia can then be topped up as and when it is needed during the labour, if its effect starts to wear off.

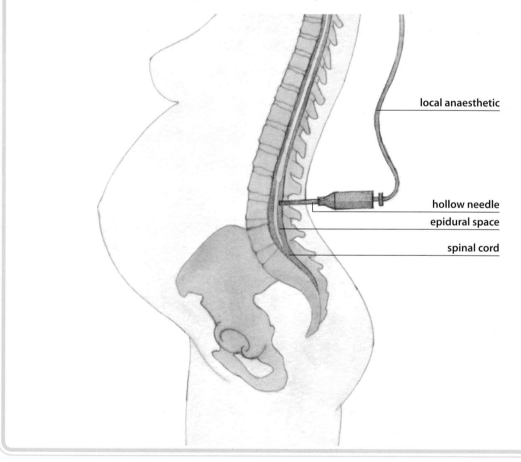

local anaesthetic

hollow needle

epidural space

spinal cord

Nitrous oxide (aka entonox, or gas and air)

This is a 1:1 mix of laughing gas and oxygen which you breath in through a mask or mouthpiece, so it's very easy to use and you can control it yourself – although if you take too much on board you may not be able to push efficiently and the midwife will try to wrestle it from you. It works really quickly (around 15 seconds), so you can suck some in with each contraction. The worst it will do, side-effects wise, is to make you feel light-headed or sick, but it's out of your system so quickly that these symptoms will pass virtually as soon as you stop using it.

Narcotics

This term is not just reserved for describing illicit drugs in US TV cop shows but is the umbrella term for morphine-like painkillers such as pethidine and, well, morphine. Pethidine is the most frequently used narcotic, as it not only works on pain but also helps ease the muscle spasms of labour. It's given as an injection into one of your muscles (usually your buttocks or thighs) and takes effect within about 20 minutes. Unfortunately it can cause quite significant nausea in around 20 per cent of women, so an anti-sickness injection often has to be given alongside it. It's effective for about three hours, but is best given in the first stage of labour as it crosses the placenta into the baby's bloodstream and can affect its breathing at birth if it is given any later. This effect can, however, be quickly reversed by giving the baby some oxygen and a dose of a drug called naloxone.

Pudendal block

The pudendal nerve is situated in the pelvis and is responsible for sensation throughout the perineum, anus, labia, clitoris and, in men, the penis. In its best moments it is responsible for the pleasure of orgasm, but when squeezed and stretched in childbirth it can transmit a fair amount of pain. Injection of local anaesthetic into this nerve (achieved by poking a needle into the vagina) will numb up this whole region of your body enough to be able to carry out forceps or ventouse deliveries and sew up vaginal tears.

Epidural or spinal block

It's probably not politically correct to call this the housewives' choice, but this type of analgesia does seem to be top of many women's lists when it comes to pain relief in labour. (See box opposite for more information on epidurals.)

Anaesthetic

In a spinal anaesthetic the injection goes into the spinal fluid itself and causes a much denser block to all nerves below the point where the injection was placed. This works more quickly than an epidural and its greater level of anaesthetic means it is sufficient to make even a Caesarean section pain-free. As for the side-effects of an epidural or a spinal anaesthetic, the most common one experienced is what's called a postdural puncture headache (PDPH) or 'spinal headache' which occurs when spinal fluid leaks out of the hole that's been made by the anaesthetist's needle. This is usually described as a severe, dull, non-throbbing pain, which is made worse when standing or sitting up but which eases when you lie down. This PDPH can often be settled simply with bed rest and plenty of fluids, but a small number of women may need to have a 'blood patch' to cure it. This involves taking a small amount of blood from a vein in your arm and injecting it back into your spine where it clots and seals up the hole.

General anaesthetic

This is reserved for emergency or 'crash' Caesarean sections, when your baby has to be delivered too quickly for you to have a spinal put in place.

Progress of labour

Once your pain relief is sorted to your satisfaction you can hopefully sit back and let the first stage of labour do its thing in reasonable comfort. Your midwife will monitor this so-called latent phase with two- to four-hourly internal examinations. The point of these is to assess the changes in your cervix (which should thin and open up at a rate of about 1 centimetre per hour) and the descent of your baby's head into the pelvis and, therefore, towards its exit.

The cervix has to 'ripen', or undergo two changes in order to allow the baby to exit via the front door: effacement (thinning out) and dilatation (opening up to a diameter of 10 centimetres). Your midwife will assess a number of features of the cervix using something known as the Bishop Score. This 'score' will give the midwife an indication of how 'ripe' the cervix is and therefore how far into labour you are. She will make this assessment by checking dilatation, length of cervix, descent of the head, consistency (firm, medium or soft – the latter being the closest to delivery) and the position of the cervix; whether it's pointing backwards, centrally or forwards (which is ideal for delivery).

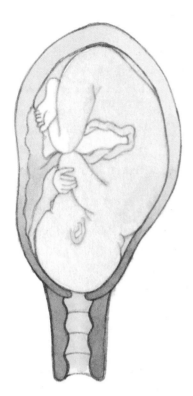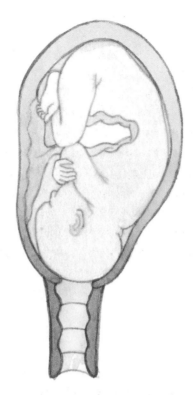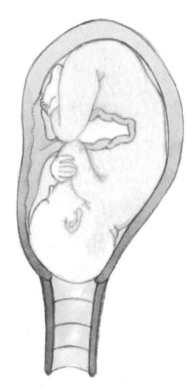

In first-timers (or primips, in medical parlance) effacement has to happen before the cervix will dilate, whereas in experienced mothers (multips) these two processes will happen simultaneously:

💧 Effacement. Throughout most pregnancies the average cervix is about 3.5 centimetres long with a very narrow canal through its centre. Nothing, least of all a baby, will pass through it. So as labour begins, some major changes have to take place in its structure to allow things to proceed. The catalyst for these changes are the prostaglandins (see above) which cause the collagen fibres (a thick connective tissue) that make up most of it structure to become weaker and come apart from each other. The cervix therefore softens, thins and re-laxes, and by the end of the process it has become an unrecognizable part of the lower end of the womb.

💧 Dilatation. As waves of contractions pass through the womb from top to bottom, the effaced cervix passively opens up and will eventually slip over your baby's head as if it was pulling on a sweater.

The descent of the head is again measured vaginally (I said there was no room for shyness in the delivery suite!) by comparing the position of your

From left to right, the cervix dilated to 2 cm, 5 cm and the final 10 cm and ready to go!

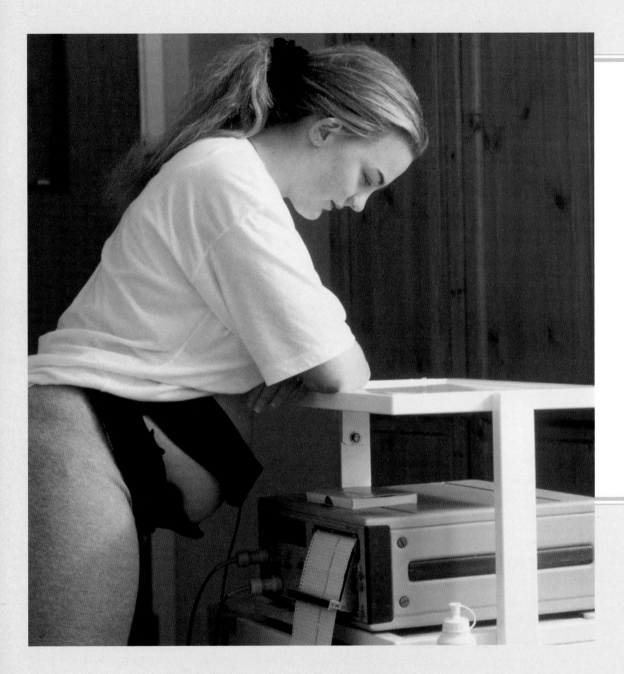

baby's head in relation to two bony prominences in the pelvis which can be felt through the vaginal wall – the ischial spines.

The level of these spines is considered as zero and the position of the head is recorded in centimetres above or below this level. So if the head is at -4 centimetres, there's a way to go yet, but at +3, it's about to make its entrance.

FOETAL MONITORING – CARDIOTOCOGRAPH

The cardiotocograph is the machine which provides the medical team looking after you with a continuous printout of both the activity of your womb and your baby's heartbeat. This, therefore, informs them how strong and frequent your contractions are (although you're unlikely to need a machine to tell you that!) and if your baby is content or struggling.

The machine is connected to you via two monitors which are held firmly to the surface of your abdomen by elastic belts. These can be disconnected from the machine from time to time to allow you to wander around, but they may become a permanent feature during the second stage if there are concerns about your baby.

Terms you might overhear about your baby's heart rate:

- Baseline heart rate: this should range between 110 and 150 beats per minute. Medics become a little twitchy if it is above or below this because it may be a sign that your baby's not getting enough oxygen (a condition known as hypoxia). It can also be caused by a fever or by various medicines.

- Variability: each beat should vary from the next by between 10 and 25 beats per minute. A loss of this variability can again suggest low oxygen or it could be caused by drugs such as pethidine.

- Dips or decelerations: this slowing of the baby's heart rate often occurs with contractions and, if so, is no cause for alarm. But decelerations occuring 15 seconds or so after a contraction are called late decelarations and these are a further sign that your baby is not getting enough oxygen and is going to be better off out of the womb.

Failure to progress in the first stage tends to be put down to a variety of things, with the reasons being classed under three headings, all beginning with the letter 'P':

- 'Power' (inadequate uterine activity).
- 'Passenger' (the baby is a whopper and too big for the pelvis or it is facing the wrong way).
- 'Passage' (the pelvis is too small).

Of course, sometimes it can be down to a combination of all three. The medical team will therefore carry out a thorough assessment of the situation based on your medical and obstetric history, the position of the baby, CTG readings, the level of descent and the degree of ripening of the cervix.

Being connected up to a cardiotocograph will allow the medical staff to keep a close eye on your baby while still in the womb.

One option that helps to get things going is to put up a drip containing a drug called oxytocin for three to four hours, as this is based on the hormone which stimulates contractions in normal labour. But for some women this solution may not be considered safe and the only option will be to perform a Caesarean section. (A Caesarean will also be needed for those women for whom oxytocin fails to move things along.)

For most women, though, the first stage eventually reaches its 'glorious' climax when the contractions become strong enough to push a baby out and the cervix is ready to provide an adequate exit. And that's when the real fun begins – in stage two!

BREECH DELIVERY

If your baby is presenting itself as breech at this stage and hasn't been picked up as such before (and somehow 10–15 per cent of babies manage to slip through the net of antenatal checks to surprise medical staff during delivery), or you have decided against a planned Caesarean, then be warned because this position will make giving birth a more risky business for the baby and can lead to trauma and asphyxia. It's also a lot more difficult to push a baby through your vagina backside first.

A large study of 2088 women carried out in 2000 by Canadian researchers came to the conclusion that Caesarean section is the safest way to deliver a baby that is breech and, as a result, most women now opt for this approach. However, in centres where they have the necessary expertise, some women still opt to have their breech babies born vaginally.

The method used to deliver breech babies naturally is very hands off (a phrase coined by British midwife Mary Cronk) and involves the baby being born using the propulsion provided by the contractions rather than by a midwife pulling on whichever bit comes out first or by using drugs to induce labour. Nevertheless, this is a procedure that you would only want carried out by the most experienced team, and if you decide to deliver this way you will have to be prepared for the possibility of an emergency Caesarean if things aren't progressing or there are potential risks for the health and safety of the baby.

Second stage labour

This stage runs from the moment your cervix is fully dilated right up to the point where your baby is delivered. Again, this part of the proceedings is divided into two phases:

Propulsive phase: This is just an extension of the first stage of labour; the head moves down through the pelvis to take up its final launch position. There may well be a lull in the contractions at this point, but it won't last for long.

Expulsive phase: This is it. The baby's head hits the pelvic floor and you get the urge to push. Now the hard work begins and it won't stop until you have a baby to show for your troubles.

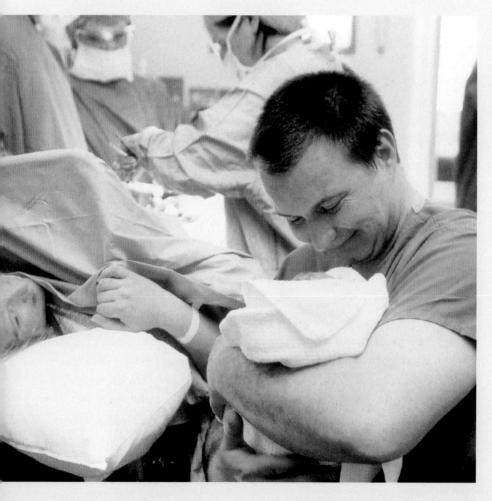

A Caesarean delivery will be recommended or even insisted upon if a baby becomes distressed during labour, or may be pre-planned in some situations, such as for babies lying breech.

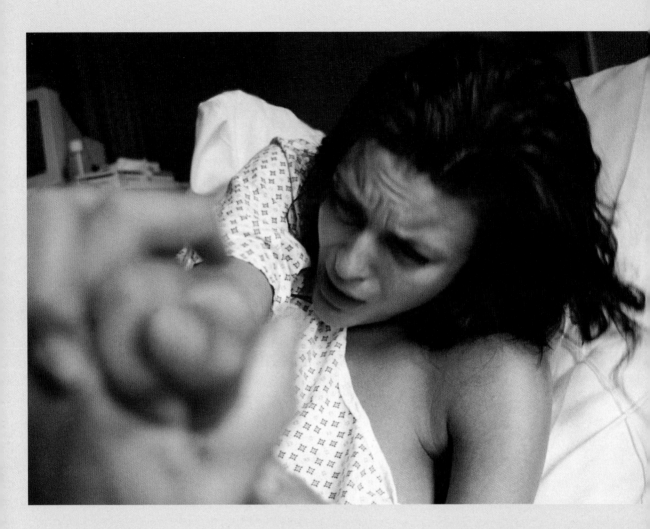

Second stage labour is when you will feel an overwhelming urge to push, and this is when you know you are nearly there!

You tend to know when the expulsive phase is about to start because you'll get an overwhelming urge to bear down and push. It is important to let your midwife guide you as to when it's best to push (during your contractions) and when it's best to get your breath back so you're ready for the next one. You don't need to go mad and strain so hard you burst a blood vessel in your forehead; just listen to your body and your midwife and you won't go far wrong.

After you've pushed your baby down through your vagina and it gets to the point where it stays there without frustratingly slipping back (and it will do that a lot during stage two), the midwife will change her tune and rather than telling you to push, she'll tell you to pant.

Panting at this point is good, because it means your baby is 'crowning' (the top of its head is visible in your vaginal opening) and if you push now the head may be propelled forwards far too quickly and tear your vagina. Many women have a weird and uncomfortable sensation down below at this point, which some people refer to as 'the ring of fire'. But pressure from the head on the vaginal nerves soon numbs the region and the sensation quickly passes.

At your next contraction you'll be asked to give a gentle push and your baby's head will be out. The midwife will then pull gently downwards to ease out the top shoulder and then pop her fingers under your baby's armpits and lift him or her up and out. The cord will then be clamped with two plastic clasps placed closely together and then be cut in the gap between the two ,either by the midwife or by your partner if that's what you prefer. (I was so overcome with the emotion of it all that the first time I tried this it took me about three attempts to get through it.)

MORE TESTS

In the first stage of labour fears about hypoxia (your baby not getting enough oxygen) may result in your baby having one of two more detailed tests – either foetal scalp monitoring or foetal blood sampling (see below) – which will be carried out to find out exactly what is happening. Neither of these tests will do your baby any harm.

In the second stage of labour a persistently worrying trace may well be the trigger for a flurry of white coats to enter your room, followed by discussions about ways to speed up delivery, such as ventouse, forceps or, in extreme cases, Caesarean section. The same may occur if the foetal scalp monitor or blood sample indicate bad news.

Foetal scalp monitoring will be carried out if the CTG reading of the baby's heart rate is not satisfactory. It involves a small clip being placed on your baby's scalp to pick up the heartbeat more directly.

Foetal blood sampling involves collecting a small drop of blood from your baby's scalp. Firstly, a tube called an amnioscope will be popped into your vagina to get a good view of its head, then some paraffin jelly is smeared on it so that the blood will collect in a blob rather than running off. A tiny nick is made in your baby's skin with a small blade and the resulting blob of blood is collected in a small capillary tube before being rushed off for analysis.

Lose your inhibitions

The second stage of labour will probably be one of the weirdest times of your life, with a whole set of sensations and emotions you've never had before rushing around your body and brain – made stranger by the fact that you may well be high on entonox or pethidine at the time.

This is the stage where you may well shout and grunt and say things you'd never dream of saying in polite company. You will probably squeeze out the odd lump of poo as you strain and if you have a hospital birth, your genitals are likely to be on display to more strangers than you'd ever wish them to be. (When we had our first baby, my wife had to put up with me, two midwives, an obstetric registrar, a medical student, a paediatric registrar and a trainee midwife all having a gawp at her privates.)

But don't be embarrassed before, during or after this stage as your midwife and medical team certainly won't be – they've seen it all before and it's all part and parcel of having a baby. Of course, by the end of labour you won't care

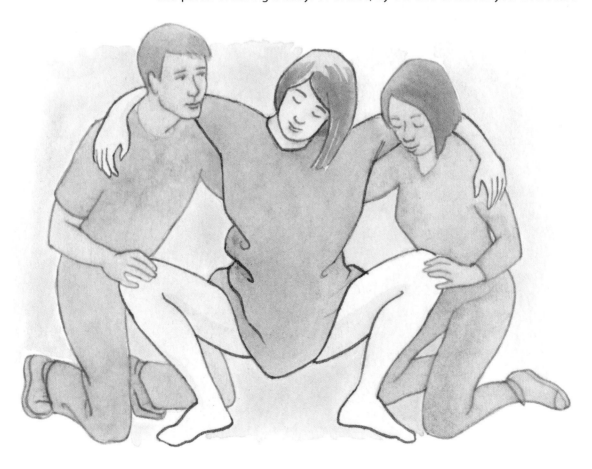

anyway, you'll just want the little perisher out and won't mind who sees where it's come from or which waste products your body expelled along the way.

And from the moment the baby's out, all that's gone before will become a distant blur. The instant you take hold of your baby and stare at its beautiful little face blinking into the light, you'll know it's all been worth it.

There's no rule that says you have to give birth lying down – unless you are hooked up to monitors. Any one of these positions might be more effective and comfortable for you.

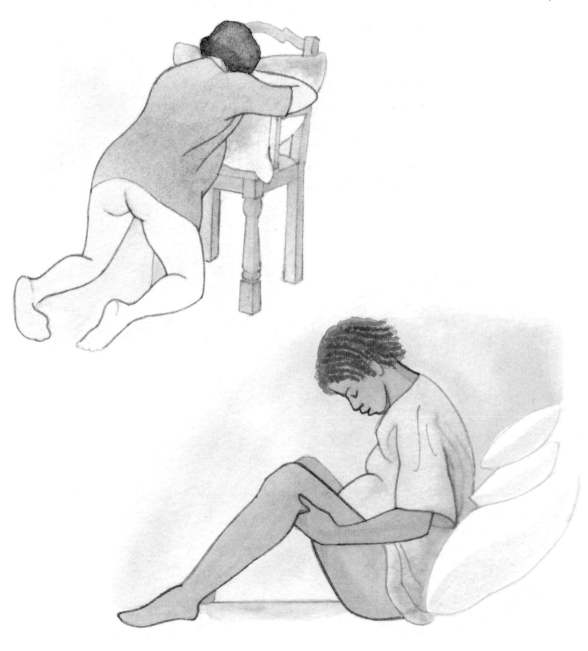

HOW YOUR INSIDES HELP YOUR BABY TO GET OUTSIDE

The inside of your pelvis is shaped rather like a funnel, but it has twists and turns in it to encourage your baby to get into the correct position for delivery. At the top, the side-to-side diameter is wider than that of front to back, whereas at the bottom of the pelvis, the dimensions are widest in the opposite direction. Hence as your baby moves downwards, he or she twists like a corkscrew so that by the time the head is as far down in the pelvis as it can go, your baby's face should be pointing towards your spine.

In this position it will be easier for the baby to duck under your pubic bone on the way out by bending its neck backwards (as you would to stoop under a low beam in a house). Some babies (including our first two) end up facing the opposite direction, which makes delivery much more difficult. This situation can be corrected by turning the baby using a ventouse or forceps.

Once the head has come through the entrance (or exit in this case) of your vagina, it will turn again and end up facing the inside of your thigh – as if it were checking your legs for cellulite. The midwife does the rest of the manoeuvring, and then – you're a mother!

1 Baby has to negotiate pelvic brim bordered by sacrum.
2 Baby moves on to pelvic outlet bordered by coccyx.
3 Contractions push baby's head down through the steepest curve at the beginning of the vagina.

Instrumental delivery

The length of your second stage will vary according to whether it's your first baby and to how well your baby behaves itself on its way out. If there are difficulties delivering the baby because of failure to progress (see page 157) or if your baby's monitor shows it's becoming hypoxic, you may need an instrumental delivery by either ventouse or forceps to help speed things up.

Ventouse

A ventouse or vacuum extractor is often brought in by a doctor during a prolonged second stage of labour or when there is foetal distress, because it is the least traumatic of the two methods for both you and your baby. It can only be used, however, if a reasonable amount of progress has been made (in other words, your baby's head is well down in your vagina), the cervix is dilated and you have sufficient pain relief on board. If you don't have an epidural then a pudendal nerve block may well be used (see page 153).

The ventouse consists of a plastic or metal cap (rather like the end of a sink plunger) which is placed on the baby's head before suction is applied. To make this easier you will have your legs lifted up in stirrups and the end of the bed will be removed so that your vagina is right up to the edge. The doctor will then check that there are no extraneous bits of your feminine parts caught underneath the cap (which would obviously give you a nasty shock when they started pulling).

Next the doctor will pull gently downwards to deliver the baby, usually with your next contraction. If you are still able to push it will obviously make things smoother. Occasionally the cap will come off your baby's head during the procedure and will simply need replacing. It won't do him or her any harm.

The ventouse cap might leave your baby with a cone-shaped lump on its head, making it look like something Doctor Who might come up against. But this is a not a serious condition and it will settle down and disappear after 24 hours or so.

Forceps

If your baby is higher up in the vagina or it needs rotating because it is facing the wrong way, the doctor may need to use forceps to get it out. These instruments come as a pair of curved blades which are joined together at a handle; this curve allows them both to fit inside your pelvis and to gently grip your baby's head.

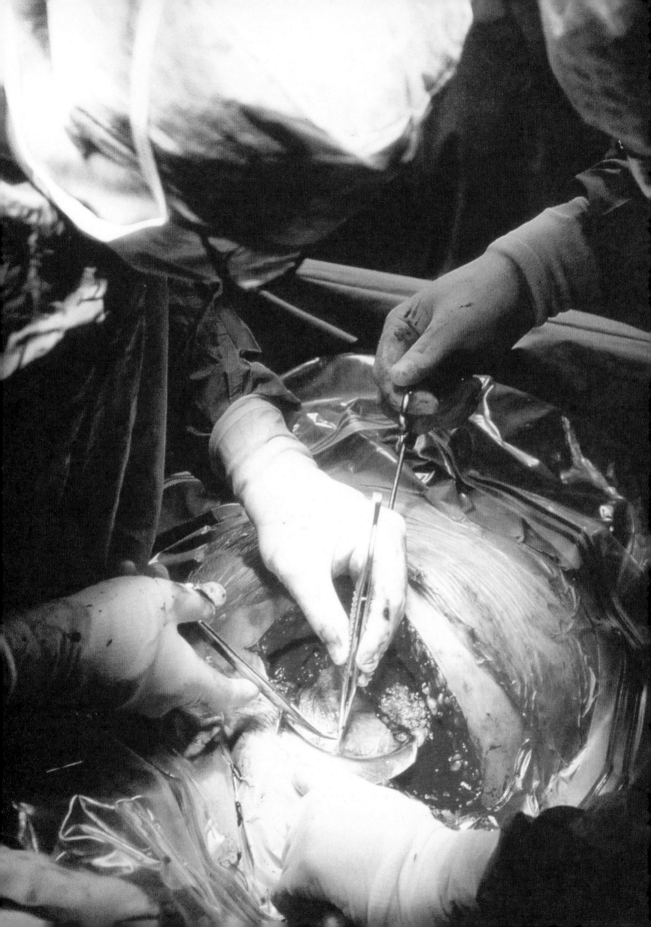

The doctor will carefully place the blades one at a time and will then use them to pull down on the baby when you push with your next contraction. They can leave marks on the side of your baby's head but, as with the bruising caused by the ventouse equipment, these will quickly fade.

Caesarean section

This method of delivery is the one that often causes controversy. On the one hand, critics feel that doctors opt for Caesareans too quickly and start sharpening their scalpels when they should be giving Mother Nature more time to do it her way. At the other end of the spectrum there are women, particularly in the entertainment industry, who seem to favour Caesarean deliveries over the normal vaginal route for vanity reasons and for convenience in their schedules.

Statistics show that around 22 per cent of British women now deliver by Caesarean section, which is roughly in line with the percentage of women having Caesareans in the United States. However, there is no indication that people in higher social classes have a more frequent rate than women in lower social classes, showing that you can never really be too posh to push.

Legend has it that Caesarean births date back to the arrival of Julius Caesar and hence the procedure took his name. But although ancient historians such as Pliny the Elder corroborate this story in their writings, it's believed by many to be just a myth, because in Roman times the procedure was solely used to deliver babies from women dying in childbirth. And Mrs Caesar was still alive when Julius was an adult.

Today, Caesareans are carried out either as elective (pre-planned) or emergency procedures. They are sometimes arranged before a woman goes into labour if the mother is suffering from placenta praevia or pre-eclampsia, is diabetic, is showing a breech presentation, if there is foetal growth restriction or because she has previously had a Caesarean and doesn't want to try to deliver vaginally. However, Caesareans are most often carried out as an emergency intervention where there is foetal distress, delay in the second stage of labour or failed instrumental delivery.

There has been an increase in the number of these operations performed each year (by a whopping 10 per cent from 12 per cent in the early 1990s), which has concerned advocates of natural childbirth. But, unfortunately, in the current climate of ambulance chasing, no-win, no-fee lawyers, many doctors are more wary of carrying out more risky procedures for fear of legal action (which accounts for 60 per cent of all payouts for medical negligence claims).

Caesarean sections are a safe way to deliver a baby in special circumstances where natural birth could cause problems for mother or baby. But it is a major operation to recover from and not the easy option.

Having had one Caesarean delivery doesn't mean that you'll have to have one next time. In fact, 80 per cent of women who delivered this way first time round will go on to have a vaginal delivery with their next child.

Third stage labour

At this point, you'll have done all the hard work; you'll have had your baby and hopefully you will now be setting about the more pleasurable business of feeding and getting to know your newborn. All that remains to be done now

WHAT HAPPENS DURING A CAESAREAN?

If it is decided that it is in your, and the baby's, best interests to have a Caesarean section, the medical staff will run through everything with you first and thoroughly explain why they have made this decision. You will then be asked to sign a consent form, to confirm that you've understood everything and are happy for them to carry on. If you don't understand something, make sure you ask the doctor to go through it again until you do. Don't worry about feeling daft – it's your body they're going to stick a knife in and you need to know exactly how and why they are going to do it.

Once the paperwork is sorted, you'll put on some rather fetching thigh-length stockings (to help prevent formation of a thrombosis in your legs) before being wheeled from your delivery room into the operating theatre. Your birth partner will have to get done up like someone out of *ER* in theatre pyjamas and a surgical hat and mask, while you'll wear a gown to keep things as sterile as possible in the operating theatre.

If you haven't had an epidural or spinal by this stage, the anaesthetist will arrange one. In a real emergency, where the baby's life may be at risk unless it's delivered immediately, you may be put to sleep with a general anaesthetic, but they'll always try to avoid this if possible.

Once you're ready a screen will be put up between your head and your belly and they will start cleaning you with antiseptic. Then the obstetrician will start by making a curved incision in the skin at near the top of your bikini line – the so-called pfannensteil

is for you to deliver the placenta, and this is known as the third stage of labour. If you are in a hospital you will now be given an injection in your leg to help this process along. (If you are having a home birth you will also be offered this injection and it's up to you whether you want to have it and speed things up, or to keep going and deliver the placenta naturally.) A drug called syntometrine is used to encourage your womb to contract and reduce the risk of bleeding. The midwife will then keep an eye on the length of umbilical cord that you'll still have protruding from your vagina. Once the placenta separates from the lining of the womb this length will increase and there will be a gush of dark blood.

incision. The layers of fat and muscle are then cut through until they reach the womb. Here, another incision will be made and your amniotic fluid will gush out everywhere (if your waters haven't already broken).

In around five minutes your baby will be out and in the arms of a paediatrician, who will check it over. Once they're happy that everything's all right, you will be able to have a cuddle with your newborn while the surgeons remove the placenta, tidy you up a bit and then sew you back up. This last bit takes a while as all the layers have to be closed up again on the way out – and that's a lot of needlework!

You will then spend some time in recovery if you've had a general anaesthetic before going back to the ward. You're likely to still have a drip going into your wrist and a tube (catheter) up into your bladder, both of which will be removed as soon as they can be. The doctors will also have popped a painkilling suppository (a drug called diclofenac) up your backside to help with pain relief in the few hours after the operation.

The midwives will have you up and about after a few hours to help reduce your risk of thrombosis, and three or four days later, once they're sure your wound is alright and your bowels are working normally, you'll be allowed home.

It is important to bear in mind that you will need some help from friends or family when you get home after this operation. It'll be another six weeks before you feel back to normal and you also won't be allowed to drive until then because the pain in your abdomen could stop you from performing an emergency stop effectively.

The midwife will then remove your placenta with what's called in the trade, 'controlled cord traction'. This is done very carefully to prevent the womb from inverting (which is the major complication).

Once it is out the midwife will check that the placenta is complete and that none of it has been left behind. She'll also have a good look at your, rather sore, vagina and labia to see if there's been any tearing. Any minor tears will be stitched up by the midwife or the junior doctor in the delivery room, with just a quick jab of local anaesthetic to numb things for you first. However, if the tear has been severe enough to reach your anus then a more senior doctor will be called in and they may need to sort things out in the operating theatre where they will have better lighting and a much clearer idea of what needs doing.

In some cases the midwife might have had to cut your perineum to help the baby out (a procedure called an episiotomy). This will again be sewn up once your placenta is out.

Your newborn baby

Once your baby has made its long-awaited entrance, your midwife will give it a quick once over to check how well it's doing in its new surroundings. This check will allow her to calculate your baby's Apgar score, which is a measure devised by an American anaesthetist (Dr Virginia Apgar) in 1953 to assess the health of babies immediately after birth.

This Agpar score is based on the observation of five factors (see table on page 172) concerning your baby and will be recorded at one minute and then five minutes after birth. The top score is a perfect ten, but anything over seven is fine. Scores of less than seven will mean that your baby will need some medical attention – such as oxygen and suction to clear secretions from its nose and mouth. Babies with scores at the lowest end of the scale may well need to be treated in the neonatal intensive care unit.

Much of this assessment can be carried out while you are holding your baby so you won't have to wait until it's finished to have a cuddle. Then, once the dust has settled and you've both had 'a moment', the midwife will clean and weigh your baby.

The medical staff will be keen to leave you to bond with your baby for as long as you like: you've already been through a lot together and will both feel exhausted and bewildered, but now is the time to begin cementing your long-awaited relationship. An early feed will help this, and if you've planned to

After your baby has been checked over, you will be left alone with it and your birthing partner to savour those first special moments and to start developing the bond that will last a lifetime.

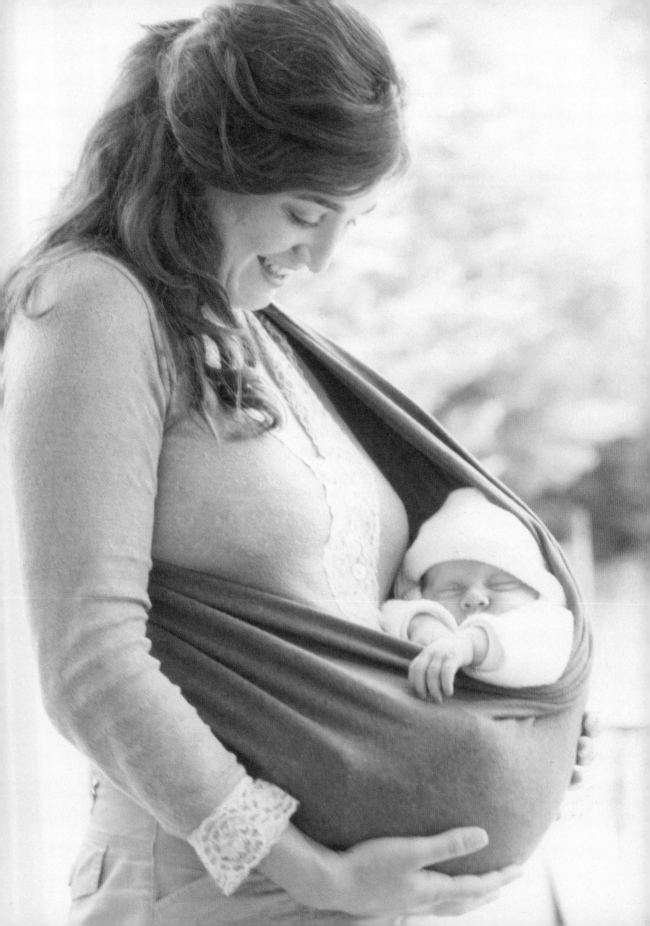

HOW TO WORK OUT YOUR BABY'S APGAR SCORE

Score	0	1	2
Heart rate	Absent	<100/minute	>100/minute
Respirations (breathing)	Absent	Slow, irregular	Good, strong cry
Muscle tone	Limp	Some flexing of arms and legs	Active motion
Colour	Completely blue or pale	Body pink with hands/feet blue	Completely pink
Reflex (response to having nose pinched)	Absent	Grimace	Grimace and cough or sneeze

breastfeed the midwife will encourage your baby to latch on to your boob as soon as possible.

Don't worry if you're unable to hold your baby straight away because the doctors are sorting either of you out or you feel too unwell, your baby won't be scarred for life as a result. In fact, we know from psychological research that bonding is a process which unfolds over weeks, not minutes, and your initial contact with your baby is only one part of this process.

Going home

If you've had a normal delivery with no complications, then after a few hours of observation (six in many units) you may well be allowed home. Obviously, if you've had a home delivery, you just stay put and the midwife leaves you, but the timescale will be similar.

Before you leave hospital, one of the paediatric doctors will do a head to foot check of your baby to confirm that all is well and may conduct a hearing test on your newborn. If you have had a home birth then this examination will be performed by your GP, who will pop in and visit you within the first 24 hours. You will be asked to attend an appointment at a later date during which the hearing test will be carried out.

Twins

When you're trying for a baby it can come as quite a shock to find out that you've been so successful in your attempts that you've actually got two on the way! For some couples twins run in the family, making it less of a surprise when this happens, while for others the news can come completely out of the blue.

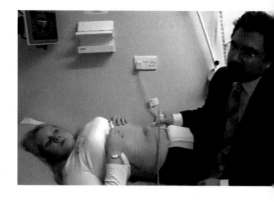

Either way, a twin pregnancy can be more problematic both antenatally and during delivery with increased risks to both mother and babies than a woman would experience with just one baby. Therefore doctors and midwives will carry out closer monitoring of mother and foetuses, meaning more appointments and scans. However this does mean that any risks are minimalized and if some are picked up then they can be dealt with quickly. As a result of this attention, most women expecting twins will have a straightforward, trouble-free time and produce healthy babies.

After a small vaginal bleed in the first few weeks, Lyndsey was sent to the early pregnancy clinic for an early scan, and it was here that she and Kevin discovered they were expecting twins. Their twins were sharing a placenta, which meant that they were monozygotic, or identical, twins.

As a result of this news and the fact that Lyndsey had had problems in her previous pregnancy (she had bleeding at 24 weeks and suffered with antenatal depression) she had intensive follow-up from the doctors with scans every two weeks throughout the pregnancy. This time, though, the pregnancy went really well and Lyndsey had no repetition of the problems she'd had last time. Closer to her due date, she was booked in to deliver the twins by Caesarean section at her local maternity unit. When the twins were born, however, it was found that one of the

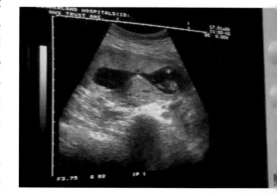

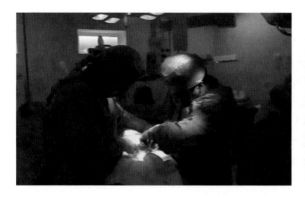
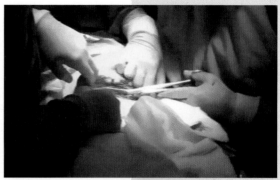
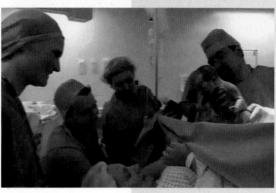

girls had a problem called a tracheo-oesophageal fistula (TOF). This rare condition occurs in around one in 3000 babies and is not exclusive to twins. This condition features an abnormal connection between the trachea (windpipe) and oesophagus (gullet) which means that food can pass into the lungs and cause choking. TOF is treated by an operation in the first few days after birth in which surgeons close off this connection. Some children can then have swallowing problems afterwards (and may need further treatment), while others will be absolutely fine.

For Lyndsey and Kevin this was obviously a tremendous shock and while they were able to take one of the twins home straight away, the other one had to stay in hospital to undergo this treatment before she too could join them back at home.

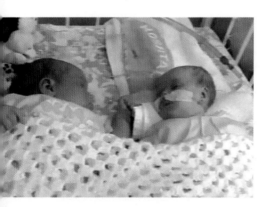

Lyndsey and Kevin's story is not, of course, common for all parents expecting twins. The majority of couples will experience no problems at all and be able to take their babies home soon after birth, so they can adapt to their new life with a house seemingly full of children and twice the normal amount of care.

It was a surprise to Lyndsey and Kevin to discover at an early scan that they were expecting twins. The pregnancy went well and the babies were born by Caesarean with Sophie delivered first and followed by her sister, Megan.

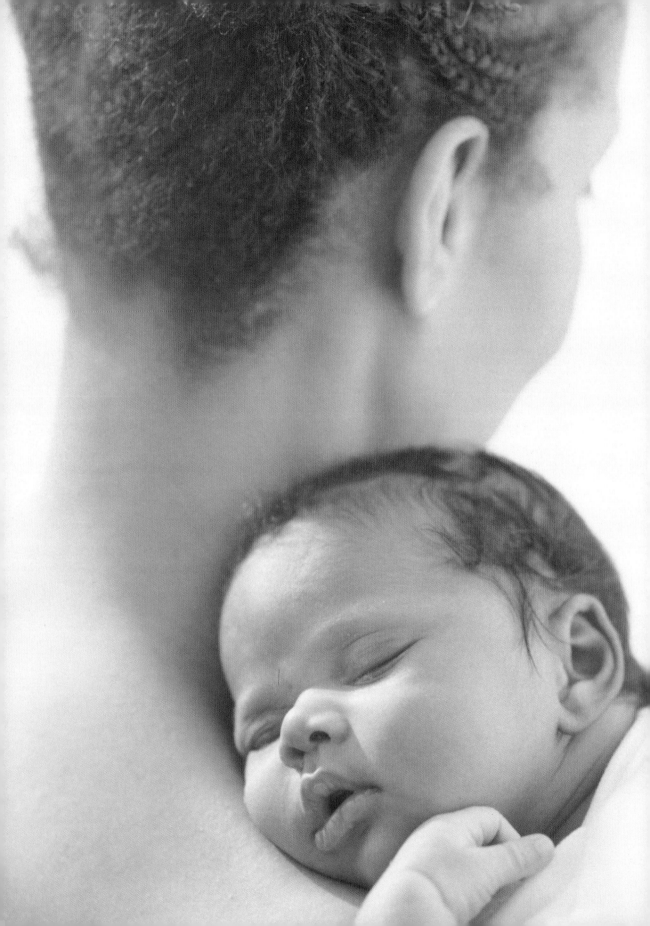

chapter 6

Coming home

Congratulations. By the time you've reached this point in the book you should be the proud owner of a brand new human being. Easy, wasn't it?

But will your life be so easy from now on? Will it be an endless round of coffee and lunch engagements where you'll show off your impeccably behaved new arrival while you relax with friends over a skinny latte and a sandwich? Or will the grim reality soon dawn on you that the devil doesn't wear Prada, he or she wears a babygro and has moved in to take over your house, your life and the hours during which you used to sleep?

Welcome to the world of parenting

For most new parents, their life has become a combination of these two scenarios – although it does get easier as time goes on, and you will eventually become a lady (or man) who lunches, if that's the lifestyle you want. But for the first few weeks, as you find your old world turned upside down, this new lifestyle can be a bit of a struggle.

You may find that you rarely get dressed until it's time to put your pyjamas on again, that your concentration and memory are shot and that you're leaking your IQ out of your boobs with your breast milk. And as for sleep deprivation, there's a reason why it has been used as a form of torture – as you'll soon discover.

No books, magazines, TV programmes or advice from well-meaning friends and family can prepare you for the adjustments you will need to make when you become parents for the first time. Babies are not predictable, and no two babies are the same or respond to the same 'rules' and routines, so not only will you need to be a natural multi-tasker, but you will also have to try to be prepared for any situation.

As junior doctors we were prey to a weird law of physics that stated that the moment a house officer closed the toilet door, their emergency pager would go off to summon them immediately to some crisis or other. The same law applies to new parents, although in their case it tends to be a high-pitched cry rather than a pager and the trigger will not just be the loo seat, but the dining room chair, the telephone and invariably your pillow.

And dads, forget any dreams of coming home to dinner on the table, a leisurely shufti through the paper and a relaxing pipe and slippers moment: it ain't gonna happen! Nor should it either. Your partner will more than likely be knackered by the time you get home (she probably was when you left) and will appreciate all the help you can give. If she hasn't been emancipated up to this point in your relationship – she will be now!

So pitch in with the chores, try your hand in the kitchen (there are plenty of blokey cookbooks out there) and take a turn with the bathing and changing. It's your baby too, and participating in those activities can help you bond with him or her, while letting your other half know how much you love and appreciate them. (See Chapter 7, page 217.)

If this new world is starting to sound a bit scary and not what you thought you were signing up for all those months ago when you saw that first peaceful scan picture of your baby, then don't panic – there's a big positive side to

There's no point in reading this section smugly if you already have kids, because even those who've been there, done that, can find adjusting to having an extra little one around just as difficult.

Second-time parents might discover that their other children's noses are put out of joint by the arrival of a new prince or princess in the family and will be treated to some right royal tantrums.

Your little angels might also exhibit some less than heavenly behaviour just to remind you that they still exist and that they still need your attention too. (A common one is to start wetting the bed again if they've previously been dry, or to start waking in the night and calling for you.)

If you've got a bigger gap between children and you're packing one or two off to school each day, you might be lucky enough to get a break while they are there, but it can be a challenge just to get to that 'quieter' part of the day.

Try doing the school run with a new baby in tow. It'll be a major achievement if you get the children there on time, dressed and armed with packed lunches, never mind being properly dressed yourself, with your milk-engorged bosoms tucked away and your hair looking slightly less deranged than an elaborate birds' nest.

So the key to survival in the early days of more than one child is organization.

Don't leave things until the last minute and always make sure that you have a contingency plan for when things slip. Make packed lunches the night before school and lay out clothes for you and your children before you go to bed to avoid a mad rush in the morning.

Do take up offers from friends and relatives to help with the school run but don't express your thanks by having too many of your children's friends home for tea just yet as it could be overwhelming. (However, always accept any offers to look after your children like a shot!)

having a new baby which makes all the hassle worthwhile. You might not think so in the early weeks, but over the following months and years they will reward you with truckloads of special moments.

If you are struggling with adapting to this demanding new lifestyle, then help is at hand in the shape of your friendly neighbourhood midwife, who'll stay in regular contact until your baby is ten days old. At this point she will pass on the baton to a health visitor, who'll also be available to give expert advice right up until your child leaves school if needs be.

If you think you are experiencing more than just baby blues, talk to any one of these health professionals, or your GP, and get some advice and support information from them. (See box on postnatal depression on pages 180–1.)

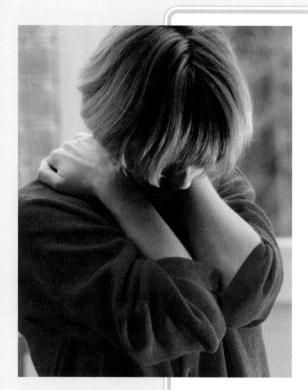

POSTNATAL DEPRESSION

It's believed that around 50 per cent of women experience some degree of 'baby blues' in the first week after giving birth (usually this happens on or around day four). This dip in mood is thought to be hormonal in origin and it can cause a variety of symptoms, including:

- Tearfulness.
- Poor sleep.
- Restlessness.
- Headaches.

For most women these symptoms disappear within a week, but in about 10 to 25 per cent of women a more severe version can occur, which usually kicks in after three to four weeks. Again, for many women, the feelings that postnatal depression can bring will soon pass on their own, but for around two-thirds of them the symptoms can become severe. In these cases the women will experience those symptoms listed above, but also might suffer from the following:

Postnatal depression is a real illness, and can take the joy out of motherhood if you don't get the help you need.

- Tiredness.
- Decreased libido.
- Inability to cope with the baby.
- Anxieties about caring for or feeding their baby.

We don't yet know what causes this condition, and in most cases it appears to be a combination of factors coming together which sets it off, such as exhaustion, a traumatic birth, a bad hospital experience, loneliness and lack of support, having a sick or premature baby, a past history of depression or a heap of life events ganging up on you at once.

So if you think you are experiencing some degree of postnatal depression it is important to get help as soon as possible. Doctors and health visitors are well trained in handling this problem and you are likely to be asked about your mood when your health visitor pops round or when you see your GP for your six-week check. Be honest in your conversations with them; they can only spot the condition and help you to overcome it if they truly know how you are feeling. You might be asked to fill out a questionnaire such as the Edinburgh Postnatal Depression Scale, which will help them to gauge the severity of your symptoms.

Postnatal depression can be successfully treated with antidepressant drugs, but counselling can also help, along with extra support from your health visitor, partner and family. You will get better but it can be a slow process, so the sooner you ask for help, the better.

You don't hear about it much, but dads can be susceptible to postnatal depression too: as many as one in 14 new fathers will develop the condition. The symptoms and treatments are the same as for women, and once again, the key advice is to seek help quickly.

PUERPERAL PSYCHOSIS

Thankfully this occurs only rarely, but puerperal psychosis is an extremely serious mental health problem which is unique to women who have just given birth. This condition affects around one or two in every thousand new mothers and usually starts in the first two weeks after having had a baby. Symptoms vary from woman to woman but will include:

- Insomnia.
- Agitation and irritability.
- Feelings of depression or being extremely happy, which can sometimes swing rapidly between the two.
- Delusions: strange beliefs that couldn't be true (often about the baby), which are held very strongly despite all evidence to the contrary.
- Seeing, hearing, touching or smeling things that aren't real.
- Confusion.
- Avoidance of the baby.

There is a very real risk that women with this condition will harm their babies, so usually they will be admitted to hospital, to mother and baby units, where they will receive medication and counselling to ensure that things improve, and where they can safely spend time with their babies to enable bonding.

Postnatal care

Much as she did with your antenatal care, soon after you've given birth your midwife will try to set out a plan of care for you and your baby so that you can both receive the support and attention that you will need at least for the first eight weeks.

The first 24 hours

Within six hours of giving birth your blood pressure will be checked, along with your urine output (if you haven't yet had a pee you may be going into retention), and you'll also be encouraged to get up and move about.

While still in the delivery suite your baby will also be offered an injection of vitamin K, which helps prevent a rare but serious blood disorder called haemorrhagic disease of the newborn. It affects less than one baby in 10,000 born in the UK, but if your baby is unfortunate enough to contract it then it can cause abnormal bleeding, particularly around the brain but also of the internal organs and the gut, and can be fatal. Vitamin K is available as an oral dose

JAUNDICE

In the first week of life around 60 per cent of full-term babies and 80 per cent of premature babies will develop a yellowish tinge to their skin. This is jaundice, which occurs when babies have too much of a chemical called bilirubin in their blood. This chemical is produced by the normal breakdown of old red blood cells and is usually removed from the body by the liver.

However, in newborns the liver takes a while to get the hang of this, hence the high levels and the yellow skin. If it is just mild and appears from around day two to day six after delivery, then it is called physiological jaundice. This is completely harmless, but your midwife will keep a watch on your baby to make sure it settles.

If, however, the jaundice is more severe, or appears at birth, then your baby may need to undergo further investigation to rule out other causes of this yellowing, such as infection, hypothyroidism (see box opposite), a liver problem or haemolytic disease.

Breastfed babies are also prone to jaundice, and the condition may hang around for two to three weeks. You are unlikely to have to stop breastfeeding but your baby may need to have a blood test to check the level of bilirubin, as severely high levels can be potentially toxic.

Treatment of these high levels usually involves phototherapy, where your baby would be put under an ultraviolet lamp. This is rarely needed, however, and in most babies the jaundice settles spontaneously.

rather than an injection if you prefer, but whichever way you choose to have it administered, it is important that your baby receives it.

In these first hours you will also be given advice on keeping baby's umbilical cord clean and about feeding – particularly breastfeeding (see page 196).

The first week

For the first week after your baby is born your midwife will stay in close contact with you and your baby. She will pay you a few visits at your home to see how you are settling in to your new life, and also to check for any symptoms of common conditions that either of you may have (see pages 190–206) and to give you any advice that you might need.

Between days five and eight the midwife will come to offer your baby the so-called heel prick test. During this quick and uncomplicated procedure the midwife will prick your baby's heel with a needle to collect a small sample of your baby's blood. She will then send off this sample to be tested for two different conditions: phenylketonuria (PKU) and hypothyroidism (see below).

WHAT THE HEEL PRICK TESTS ARE FOR

Phenylketonuria (PKU) is a rare, inherited disorder in which there is a build up of an amino acid in the blood (part of a protein molecule) called phenylalanine.

This amino acid is found in a number of foods, including meat, cheese, poultry, eggs and milk, and if a child with this condition has these foods then the level of phenylalanine will build up to a dangerous level because their body lacks the enzyme needed to break it down.

This in turn causes learning disabilities and epilepsy.

If the PKU disorder is picked up early then it can be treated very easily simply by avoiding foods which contain this amino acid. So babies who are identified as having PKU as a result of the heel prick test will be put on a special diet for life.

Hypothyroidism is another condition that affects a baby for life. The thyroid gland, from which this condition gets its name, is a lump at the front of the neck which releases a

hormone called thyroxine into the bloodstream. Thyroxine has an important role in the control of growth and metabolism, and if the thyroid gland fails to produce enough of it (or if the gland is missing altogether), babies can suffer developmental abnormalities which will cause growth restriction and learning disabilities.

Hypothyroidism is treated with a lifelong course of medication which is designed to replace the missing hormone, and it does so very effectively.

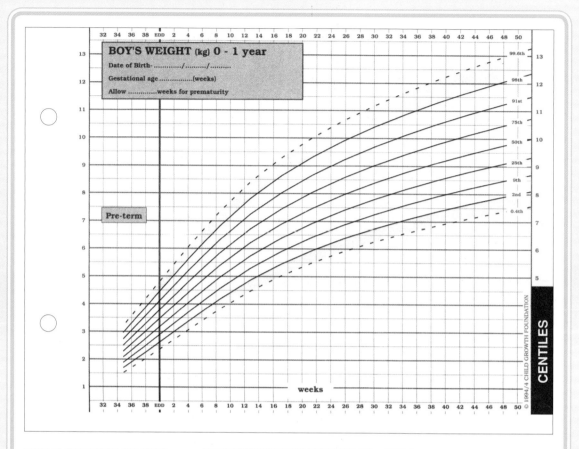

CENTILES

DEVELOPMENT CHARTS

Once your baby is registered with a doctor, the health visitor will give you a red book in which the outcome of all your visits to health professionals will be documented. This will involve recording every vaccination that is given. They will also use various charts to plot your baby's weight and height so you can make sure he or she is growing well.

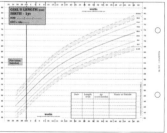

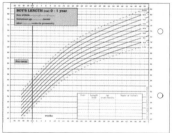

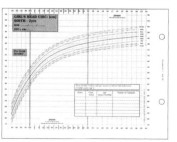

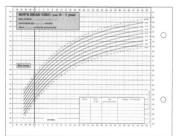

The first two months

After ten days your care will be handed over to a health visitor, who will stay in touch as your child grows to help with any problems. They will also perform tests such as a hearing test (although some hospitals now carry out this test before your baby goes home).

The Otoacoustic Emissions Test, or hearing test, involves placing a small soft-tipped ear piece in the outer part of your baby's ear, which emits clicking sounds. When an ear receives sound the inner part, known as the cochlea, usually produces an echo. Using a computer, the tester can see whether this echo occurs in response to the clicks and therefore if your baby's hearing is okay. It only takes a few minutes and you stay with your baby while the test is done. Even more reassuringly, you'll get the results straight away.

If this test shows a poor response, it doesn't necessarily mean that your baby will have hearing problems, but you will be asked to attend further tests to make sure all is well.

The six-week check

At around the six-week mark, you (rather than your baby) will be offered a check-up with your doctor to make sure that everything's gone back to normal for you and your body after having your baby.

Doctors won't routinely do an internal examination these days, unless you are concerned about a specific problem, but they'll check your blood pressure and have a general chat to you about life as a mum, to make sure you're not showing any signs of postnatal depression (see pages 180–81). They'll also discuss contraception with you, as it's possible to conceive again frighteningly quickly after having a baby!

The eight-week check

This check is for your baby and involves a top to tail once-over by a doctor and a series of questions for you to make sure you're happy with the way your baby responds to you and the world around them. The doctor will check your baby's eyes, mouth, heart, lungs, abdomen, hips (see box on page 186) and their fontanelles (soft spots at the front of their skull), and they will be weighed and measured. They'll also check to see if a boy's testicles have both dropped.

Next the doctor will test a number of simple reflexes to make sure your baby's nervous system is working properly. One of these, the Moro or startle reflex, looks a bit cruel, but don't worry, it isn't. The doctor will lift your baby up from a lying position with its head supported by one hand, then the head will be dropped back suddenly (just a few centimetres!) and quickly caught again. If the nervous system is developing normally, then your baby's arms will be thrown straight out at the sides in a startle response.

At this appointment the doctor will also check your baby's finger grip, whether he or she has good head control and that he or she isn't too floppy.

Once the examination is over, your baby will have its first set of jabs (or you might be asked to make an appointment with the practice nurse for these) and then you're done.

CONGENITAL HIP DISLOCATION

Congenital dislocation of the hip is a condition in which the ball of the baby's thigh bone becomes dislodged from its socket in the hip bone. It's not painful, so unless the baby is examined specifically for dislocation (as it is at the postnatal check) it won't show up until the child starts to walk, when they will demonstrate a limp, and they will later be at risk of developing arthritis.

If this condition is picked up early, however, most babies can be successfully treated using a special splint which holds the hip in its socket. Occasionally an anaesthetic might be needed to replace the hip, after which a baby is put into a frog plaster (which holds their legs in a position a bit like a frog's). In rare cases where this treatment does not work, or where the dislocation is found late, an operation might be needed to correct things, after which the child will have to spend the next six months in plaster.

Immunizations

New babies will be given their first set of vaccinations at their eight-week check (or thereabouts if the doctor refers you to the nurse for this), and this is followed up by two more 'booster' sets, each given one month apart.

Vaccinations are a controversial part of parenting, but they are undoubtedly very effective in protecting against serious illnesses.

Immunization of children has caused a lot of controversy since the MMR scare first hit the front pages in 1998, but since then a lot of research has been carried out into the safety of this and other vaccines and no link has been found between these immunizations and longer term health problems (in particular between MMR and autism). In fact, since the scare a number of parents have

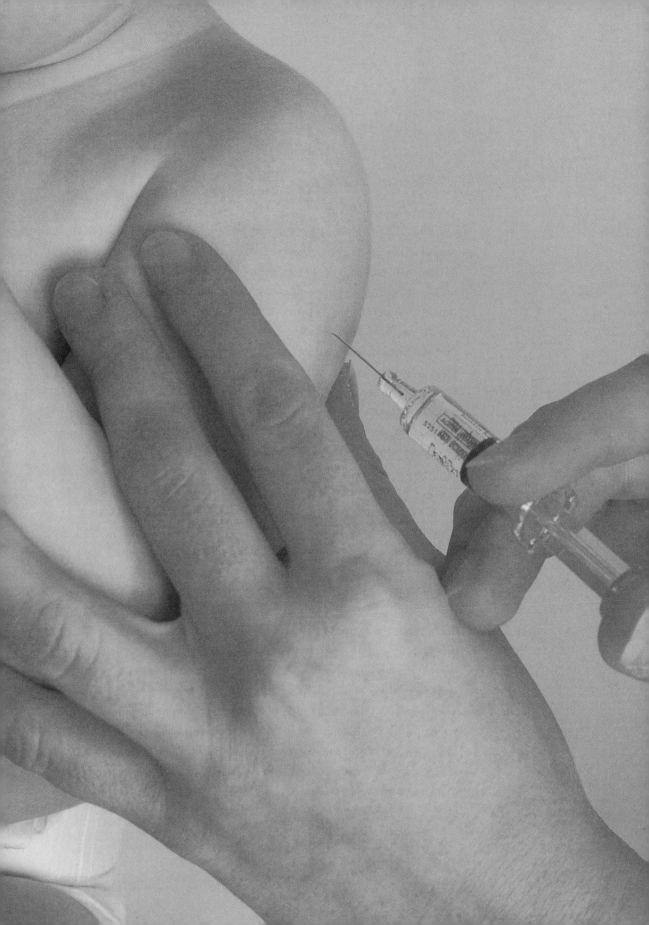

stopped vaccinating their children against various diseases and this has led to outbreaks of the conditions they are designed to prevent (some of which have life-threatening consequences). This in itself serves to underline the importance of having your children protected by vaccination.

HOW VACCINES WORK

The term vaccination was first coined by Gloucestershire doctor Edward Jenner in 1796, when he noticed that milkmaids who had had a dose of cowpox (a much milder illness) seemed not to catch the potentially lethal smallpox which was rampant at the time (*vacca* comes from the Latin word for cow). To prove that cowpox had a protective effect against smallpox, he injected some cells from a cowpox blister on a milkmaid, called Sarah Nelmes, into an eight-year-old boy, called James Phipps. He then gave the boy a mild dose of smallpox and (I'm sure to his great relief) James didn't pick up the infection, demonstrating that vaccination was effective.

Vaccines work on the body's immune system, which is designed to protect us against infection. There are two types of immunity:

- Active immunity: this protection is produced by our own immune systems when they recognize invading micro-organisms and trigger the production of chemicals to destroy them, called antibodies, and white blood cells called lymphocytes.
- Passive immunity: this protection is provided by someone else's immune system, most commonly when a mother's antibodies pass from the placenta into her baby.

Vaccines are made from killed organisms – live organisms that have been inactivated – or parts of their outer cell walls. All of these will contain the key identifying factors for that bug, which our immune systems will then remember.

The vaccines stimulate active immunity by provoking the immune system with a small sample of an infectious organism, which it will then recognize and kill if it comes across it again. It's a bit like letting a police sniffer dog smell an item of someone's clothing so that they can track them down and catch them.

Many parents fear that all the jabs that children are now expected to have are too much for their young immune systems. But we are exposed to thousands of germs in our environment every day, so a child's system can easily cope with a few extra. And rather than being overwhelming, these injections help to provoke their immune systems into action.

VACCINE SCHEDULE IN THE FIRST YEAR

8 weeks

Diphtheria, tetanus, pertussis (whooping cough), polio and *Haemophilus influenzae* **type b (Hib) (DTaP/IPV/Hib). One injection.**
Pneumococcal infection (Pneumococcal conjugate vaccine, PCV). One injection.

12 weeks

Diphtheria, tetanus, pertussis, polio and *Haemophilus influenzae* **type b (Hib) (DTaP/IPV/Hib). One injection.**
Meningitis C (meningococcal group C) (MenC). One injection.

16 weeks

Diphtheria, tetanus, pertussis, polio and *Haemophilus influenzae* **type b (Hib) (DTaP/IPV/Hib). One injection.**
Meningitis C (meningococcal group C) (MenC). One injection.
Pneumococcal infection (Pneumococcal conjugate vaccine, PCV). One injection.

Around 12 months old

Haemophilus influenzae **type b (Hib) and meningitis C (Hib/MenC). One injection.**

For more information on each of these individual vaccines you can speak to your doctor or health visitor, or visit the NHS vaccination website, at www.immunisation.org.uk

Vaccinations are offered to help your child to stay healthy and happy, but if you have any concerns, do discuss them with your doctor.

Common postnatal problems (mother)

It takes around six weeks after giving birth for your body to return to the way it was before you became pregnant – although this may take longer for some parts than others (such as losing that extra baby weight, for example). Your body has been through an incredible experience over the last nine months and so, inevitably, it has a few major adjustments to make to go back to its previous way of functioning, now that the baby-making job is done.

Of course, this can cause you to experience a few strange sensations over the next few weeks and months. Most of the time you'll have a trouble-free recovery but your body can put an odd spanner in its works.

Involution of the womb

This is the technical way of describing the process during which your womb contracts from its enlarged state just after delivery (when it weighs about 1kg) to its pre-pregnancy size and weight of around 80g.

Your womb will reduce in size reasonably quickly, so that by the time you've had your baby it will already be down by your belly button, and within two weeks it will have shrunk right down below the pelvic brim and won't be able to be felt at all. At the same time, the muscle cells in the wall of the womb will break down, reducing them to being simply protein molecules which then pass into the bloodstream before being removed from your body in your urine.

This whole process is sped up by breastfeeding and slowed down by having a full bladder, being constipated or if there are any remnants of your placenta left behind after delivery.

After two weeks your cervix will also have closed and by week three after birth your vagina will be back to its normal shape and size.

Menstruation

If you are not breastfeeding your baby, then after three weeks your womb will create a new lining and so you will usually have your first period by about six weeks.

It doesn't take a genius to work out that if this is happening, then you are fertile again and could potentially conceive another baby very soon after having your last. This is why your midwife and doctor will discuss contraception with you at around the time of your six-week check. (I have a few patients with children who are only ten months apart, so it's worth taking this part of the appointment seriously.)

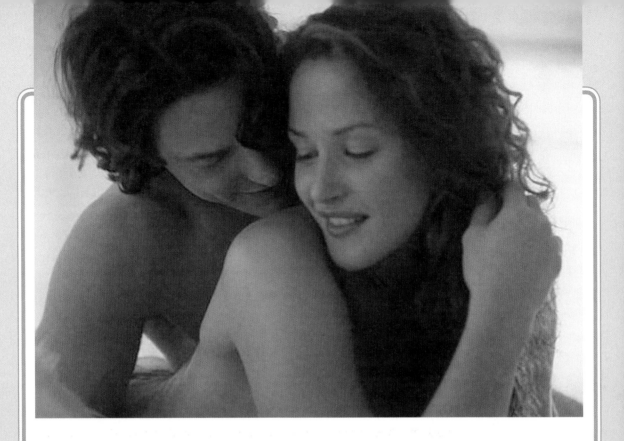

SEX AFTER CHILDBIRTH

Once your doctor or midwife has told you that everything has healed up down there, then it's quite safe to have sex.

However, given all the symptoms of perineal pain, lochia, breast soreness and general tiredness, it's quite natural that returning to having sex with your partner is the last thing on your mind.

To avoid frustration and the feeling of being under pressure to 'perform', it's a good idea to talk to your partner about how you're feeling with regards to resuming your sex life. If you're not ready yet, don't discount intimacy altogether: it's amazing how beneficial a good cuddle can be. Once your sex drive has returned, it's best to take things steady to begin with. Your bits and pieces may well feel a bit different at first, particularly if there are scars from stitches, and you might find using a lubricant jelly will help.

If you are breastfeeding your baby, then your body's hormones will inhibit the menstrual cycle to an extent and you may not have a period until you stop feeding. However, and it's a big however, you may still be ovulating – which means that you can still get pregnant. So don't trust your breasts to take care of your contraceptive needs. You might be advised to go on the mini pill (which is safe when breastfeeding), to have a coil fitted, or to use condoms, so as to avoid hearing the patter of more tiny feet too soon.

Lochia

This is the name given to the blood-stained vaginal discharge which you will have after giving birth. It will usually fade to a pinky colour after a few days, becoming clear after a week or so. However, if it stays red you should ask your healthcare professional about it as you might have an infection or some placenta left behind in your uterus. If the discharge is smelly and you feel feverish and unwell with some abdominal pains, then it is very likely that you have an infection and you may need a trip to hospital to be put on intravenous antibiotics to settle it down.

The midwife and health visitor will monitor this, so do mention anything you are concerned about to help them, and you, to pick up any problems early on.

Some potential problems for new mothers

After the battering your body has been exposed to, it's unlikely to come as a surprise that you might now experience the odd twinge here and there. There is also the possibility of the odd complication caused by having your figure stretched out of proportion and all your bodily systems rearranged. For most women these problems are at worst mild, but there are a few more severe ones worth keeping an eye out for.

Deep vein thrombosis

Deep vein thrombosis is not a disorder that is exclusive to people flying economy class on airlines; it can also occur after you've had a baby – especially if it was delivered by Caesarean section.

The actual thrombosis occurs when a blood clot forms inside one of the deeper veins of the body, and most commonly this is in the legs. This clot will disrupt your body's blood circulation and, at worst, pieces can break off and travel through the bloodstream in a process called embolization. Eventually these so-called emboli become blocked as the blood vessels narrow in places like the lung or brain and can cause severe damage, or even death.

Symptoms of a thrombosis in the leg usually arise first in the calf muscles and include:

- Muscle pain.
- Swelling of the lower leg.
- Skin redness.

If you get this set of symptoms then you need to be checked over by your doctor straight away. If they're accompanied by shortness of breath and pain in the chest then you need to call an ambulance and get over to the accident and emergency department of your nearest hospital.

If a clot is suspected then you'll need a blood test and leg or chest scan to confirm things, after which proven thromboses will be treated with blood thinning injections and then three to six months of warfarin tablets to dissolve the clot.

Perineal pain

The perineum is, as we've already discovered, the technical name for the part of your body located between your vagina and anus. Obviously this part of your anatomy gets quite a hammering during a vaginal delivery, so it's not really surprising that 40 per cent of women who give birth naturally and 80 per cent of those who have an instrumental delivery will have perineal pain postnatally; and this can last for up to two months.

Simple treatments such as ice packs, local anaesthetic creams and anti-inflammatory suppositories prescribed by your doctor can help, and some women swear by the homoeopathic remedy arnica (although the evidence that these tablets are much better than sugar pills is slim). Occasionally women are referred to physiotherapists for ultrasound treatment of perineal pain but, again, the evidence for its effectiveness seems to be weak.

If pain is associated with fever and any sign of pus, then it is likely to mean there's an infection, and if so your doctor may need to send you back to the maternity unit for a course of intravenous antibiotics.

Bladder problems

There are whole textbooks' worth of problems that can impact on the normal functioning of the bladder after you have had a baby. Many women find they have trouble 'going' because of the effects of an epidural or a spinal anaesthetic, perineal pain, or because they are constipated. For others the problem might be the reverse and they might suffer incontinence. It's not too late to do your pelvic floor exercises now to help this (see page 121).

It is also common for women to pick up urinary tract infections, such as cystitis, after delivery. Such conditions make it painful to pee, give you a fever and will make you go to the loo a lot, only to pass very small quantities when you get there. If you are suffering from a 'uti', then you will be asked to send a urine sample for testing and you might be given some antibiotics to settle it down.

Bowel problems

Again, women can be haunted by the twin spectres of having trouble going and having trouble holding on. Constipation is a really common problem for new mothers, and one that is made worse by the fear of aggravating perineal pain or causing haemorrhoids to bleed by having your bowels open.

The key here is to drink plenty of water and eat platefuls of fruit and veg to keep things soft and easy to pass. If it all gets a bit ridiculous and you've not had a turn out for days, your doctor can prescribe laxatives to get things moving again. Bowel incontinence always requires a medical check-up, as more detailed investigation of your sphincter function may be needed. Pelvic floor exercises can certainly help reduce the risk of this.

Breast problems

Around two-thirds of breastfeeding women will experience problems with sore, cracked nipples, bleeding, painful engorgement and mastitis. Advice about better positioning of the baby can help prevent many of these symptoms, but once they occur then you need to apply one of a variety of creams, such as lanolin or camomile based kamilosan, that are available over the counter. Breastmilk itself is also believed to have a soothing effect.

If your baby has thrush in its mouth (which can usually be seen as a white coating on the tongue, the roof of the mouth and inside the cheeks), then this may be responsible for your sore nipples. Make an appointment to see your midwife or health visitor, who may well advise you to get a prescription from your doctor to clear things up for both of you.

Mastitis is a condition which results in inflammation of one or both breasts and is usually caused by infection from a skin bacterium called *Staphylococcus aureus*. This infection causes redness, swelling and hardening of the affected breast, along with pain, a high fever and a general feeling of crappiness. It can be treated successfully with antibiotics, although hot showers or hot compresses can also help to relieve the pain until the drugs kick in, along with paracetamol and (apparently) by popping the chilled leaves of a savoy cabbage inside your bra. Experts suggest that you should continue breastfeeding on the affected side, as this will help to relieve the mastitis without harming the baby. Your doctor will make sure that any antibiotics prescribed are safe for breastfeeding mothers too.

TOP TIPS FOR POSTNATAL SURVIVAL

◊ If friends or relatives offer help with cooking, cleaning, ironing, or anything really, accept it gratefully!

◊ If you have a choice between doing the chores and sleeping, then sleep.

◊ Aim to get out of the house every day; a bit of fresh air will be good for both of you.

◊ Find some adult company and share your worries and concerns with friends rather than bottling it all up.

◊ Make time to go out alone with your partner and don't be afraid to use trusted babysitters.

◊ Do your pelvic floor exercises.

◊ Make sure you eat a decent balanced diet at regular times during the day and try to drink plenty of fluids, especially if you are breastfeeding.

◊ Join a parent and baby group to catch up with other new mums.

◊ If you have other children, have their packed lunches sorted and their clothes laid out ready the night before, to save on early morning crises.

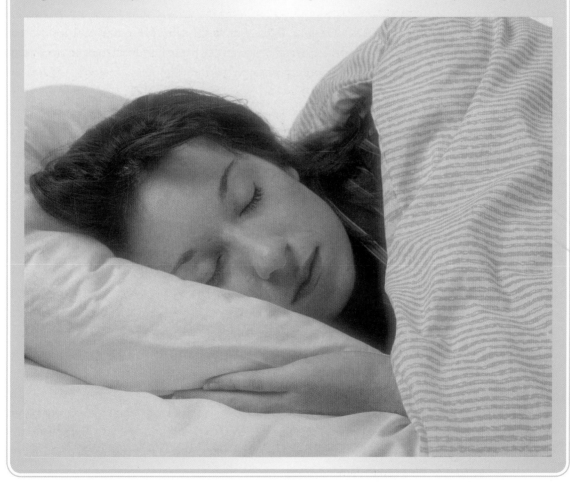

Feeding

Newborn babies have a pretty simple diet, consisting of milk washed down with a nice drop of milk, and they can't take solid food until they're around six months old. That may seem like an obvious statement, but having heard from a health visitor how a young mum she once knew used to chew up chips to regurgitate into her baby's mouth, it's probably worth mentioning…

Baby's milk can come in two forms, and it's up to you which one you use:
- Formula, which is manufactured in factories.
- Breastmilk, which is manufactured in your, er, breasts.

As a doctor, you might think I'm bound by the Hippocratic oath to say that breast is best when it comes to feeding your baby, but there's no official arm-twisting or threats from on high when it comes to dishing out this advice. It's simply true. And despite all the technology available to the manufacturers of formula milk, nothing else can replicate all of the goodness that Mother Nature has bottled up in a woman's bosom.

Breastfeeding

The World Health Organization recommends that babies should be breastfed for the first six months of their life but, although in the UK around 71 per cent of mothers will start to feed their babies this way, by the end of the first week only 57 per cent are still at it, and by six weeks that figure has dropped to just 43 per cent.

That said, there will, of course, be some women for whom breastfeeding presents so many problems that the bottle is the only available option – and it will do the job fine. But if you *can* give it a go on the breast (and let's be honest, the vast majority of women and their babies are physically able to), then it is well worth having a try.

Unfortunately, despite all of the evidence about its inherent benefits, breastfeeding literally gets a bad press. In a study in the *British Medical Journal* in 2000, researchers found that media coverage of infant feeding was far more likely to feature the use of bottles than boobs, and indeed it rarely presented any positive information about breastfeeding. In fact, the take-home message seemed to be that bottle-feeding was easier and was the normal thing to do for ordinary families.

When it comes to nurturing your newborn, breast is best – and for those who aren't keen, remember that even a few weeks of mother's milk can be beneficial.

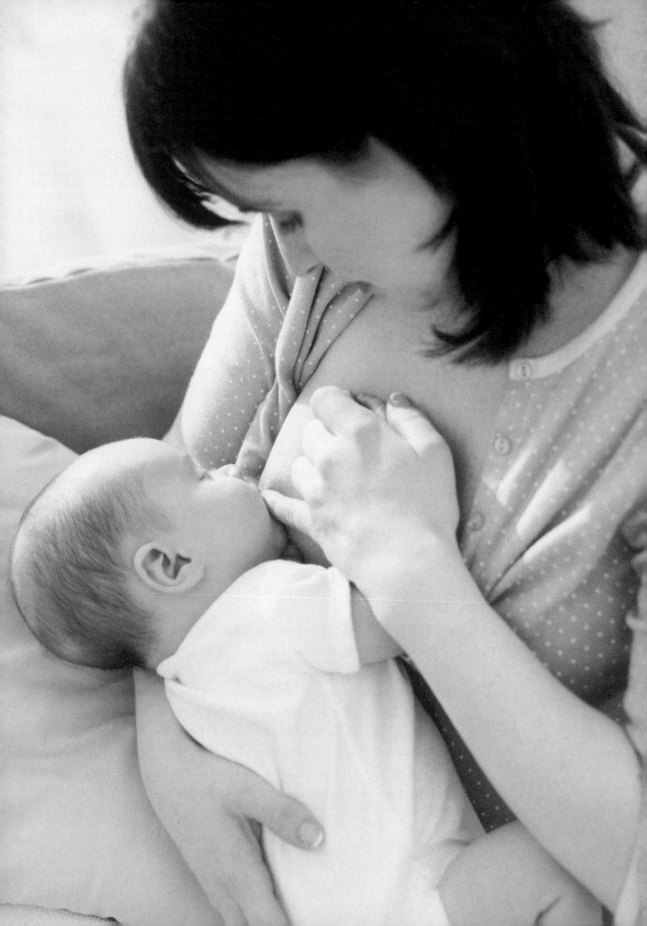

Of course that's nonsense, and once you've got the hang of breastfeeding it's the most convenient way of feeding there is. Nothing needs sterilizing; it comes out at the right temperature; and it's free.

Although breastfeeding appears to be more common among women in the so-called middle class, it certainly shouldn't stay that way. All breast milk is created equal: don't let embarrassment get in the way of the best start in life that your baby can have. It is possible to get your breasts out in public without looking like a wannabe stripper on a stag night. Nursing bras allow undressing to be very discreet and there are a number of shopping centres that have rooms where you can feed your baby in private, if you prefer. But if you want to just lob them out, then why not? If more women just got on and did it, it would be far less of a big deal in the first place.

ADVANTAGES OF BREASTFEEDING FOR YOUR BABY

- The skin-to-skin contact helps them to bond with you quickly.
- Breastmilk contains immunoglobulins and germ-busting cells (called macrophages) which pass over from your bloodstream and help to protect your baby against infections.
- They are less likely to pick up ear infections, urinary tract infections, chest infections and gastroenteritis than bottle-fed babies.
- Breastmilk protects your growing baby against the development of allergies, asthma and eczema.
- Breastfed babies suffer constipation less than bottle-fed babies.
- Breastmilk seems to reduce the risk of children developing diabetes.

ADVANTAGES OF BREASTFEEDING FOR YOU

- It may decrease your chances of getting breast cancer, ovarian cancer and osteoporosis.
- It stimulates the production of the hormone oxytocin, which helps your womb to return to its normal size after delivery, and it also helps you to return to your previous size by ridding you of the extra pounds you stored up during pregnancy.
- You may not have any periods until you stop feeding, although do not rely on this as a method of contraception.

Mother's milk

For a few days after giving birth a thick, sticky, golden-yellow liquid called co-lostrum will be on the menu for your baby. This milk is packed with proteins, carbohydrates and antibodies and serves as an excellent, nutritious first food.

At around three or four days after delivery your milk 'comes in' and you start producing larger volumes of the thinner, whiter liquid that you will make until you stop breastfeeding. At this time your breasts will also become bigger and harder, and they can feel quite uncomfortable until the baby starts to feed enough to relieve this engorgement. (They may also not behave themselves and can leak the stuff out at the sound of your baby's cry – and during orgasm – so have your breast pads at the ready, and warn your partner that during sex things can get a little interesting!)

Ask your midwife for advice on getting breastfeeding going, or call one of the support groups listed at the end of the book.

Technique

You both need to be comfortable and relaxed, so put the answerphone on and find a quiet, relaxing spot (although if you have other young children charging around, good luck to you!):

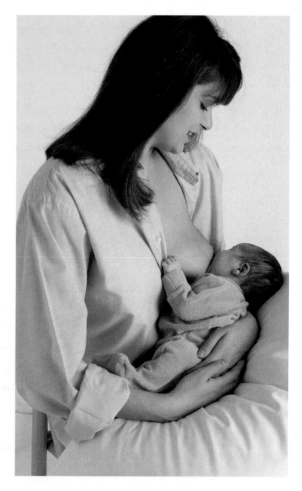

- Sit with your back straight and a flat lap and put a pillow on it to support your baby.
- Hold your baby so that their tummy is towards you (apparently 'tummy to mummy' is the very twee way to remember it).
- Tuck your baby's bottom under your elbow and, holding them behind their neck and shoulders, line up their nose with your nipple.
- Allow their head to tip back and as you move their mouth gently across your nipple it should open wide. At this point pull them quickly towards your nipple so that they can attach themselves (or 'latch on') and start feeding.

You may need to support your breast with your other hand, but you can usually move this away once feeding has started.

All this may take time to perfect but you'll get there – and don't be afraid to ask the midwife for help.

Formula feeding

Formula milk is based on cow's milk and, although it doesn't give the same protection as breast milk, it does contain all the correct nutrition a baby needs in the first six months.

Make sure you follow the instructions on the pack carefully when making up formula milk, as too much, or too little, could be harmful to your baby. If you are warming bottles then you need to check the temperature of the milk is not too hot before feeding it to your baby.

Formula has come on in leaps and bounds in recent years and contains all the right stuff for a growing baby.

For convenience you can make up feeds for the whole day and store them in the fridge, but you should tip them away if they've not been used within 24 hours. Or you can fill bottles with water and measure out the powder into a dispenser (which are widely available), so you need only make up the bottles as and when you need them, sparing wastage.

You will also need to pay particular attention to hygiene when preparing bottles and ensure that all feeding equipment is completely sterilized at least for the first six months to a year. There are a number of sterilizers on the market to help with this.

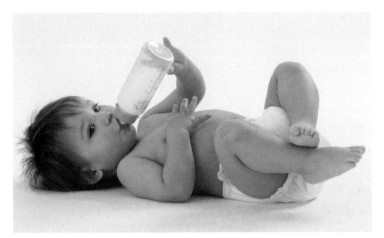

Potential problems for newborn babies

Becoming a parent brings with it a life of worry about your children and of being in uncharted waters. Be assured, though, that most of the time your baby will be absolutely fine and there is no need to be concerned. However, every now and then children are prone to various blotches and rashes and the odd disruptive outburst.

Here's a troubleshooting guide to some of the most common problems they might encounter in the early days.

The skin

Very little babies can get a few different rashes, most of which are nothing to worry about, but it's worth mentioning them here, if only for reassurance should you see them.

Erythema toxicum

This is a lot less nasty than its name suggests and is a common rash that nearly all babies will have in the first week of life. It consists of red spots with white heads on them which can appear anywhere on a baby's body.

It causes no harm whatsoever, doesn't need treating and goes away on its own. I probably see a new baby every month or so with this rash in surgery and I can always reassure mums that their babies are fine.

Milk spots (milia)

These are also very common and are found on around 50 per cent of new babies. They are seen as white spots on the nose and cheeks and, again, they will disappear spontaneously.

Stork bite

This is technically known as a capillary haemangioma and can be found on the eyelids, nose, upper lip and the neck in around half of newborns. These marks are caused by distended capillaries (the small blood vessels under the skin) and usually clear up by the time a baby is one year old. However, sometimes this mark holds its ground when it appears on the neck, but it won't cause any problems even if it never fades.

Other 'birth marks' may well be more permanent and may need referral by your doctor to a plastic surgeon for cosmetic treatment. If you are concerned about a mark, see your doctor for advice.

Sucking pad

This is a dry thickening on the upper lip which is caused by repeated sucking, much like getting a blister if your shoe rubs. No treatment is required and they vanish spontaneously.

Nappy rash

This will appear after prolonged contact between your baby's skin and wee and poo in their nappies. It usually causes a bright red rash on the buttocks, upper thighs and around their genital area, but it tends not to affect the creases.

One of the key measures to help prevent and treat this condition is simply to change their nappies frequently. But barrier creams such as Sudocrem and moisturizers such as E45 can also help. If these don't clear it up completely then it may be that there's a thrush infection on your baby's skin, in which case your GP can prescribe an antifungal cream to finish off the job.

Hormonal symptoms

Breast enlargement

Both baby boys and girls can have enlargement of their breasts in the first two weeks after birth. Occasionally these breasts will also produce milk, often known as 'Witches Milk'.

Although both of these breast symptoms can cause alarm, neither are serious; they are both simply the result of the female hormones (particularly oestrogen) that the baby picked up in the womb still whizzing around its system.

The hormones will disappear within the first two weeks after delivery, and so will the breasts and the milk.

Vagina

Some baby girls will have a whitish vaginal discharge soon after birth which can be tinged with blood. Their mother's hormones are again the culprits and the symptoms will settle once these hormone levels have dropped.

Umbilicus

After the cord has been cut your baby will have a short strand of its umbilical cord stuck to its belly button. Initially this will look creamy coloured and feel rubbery, but after a while it will dry out and look black and wizened, and it will then drop off after a week or so.

It's quite safe to bath your baby while it still has this stump, but do keep an eye out for infection as this may need some antibiotics to settle it. Signs of infection would include reddened skin around the stump and foul smelling pus coming from underneath it.

Occasionally when the cord has dropped off a baby is left with a bright red area of skin in its belly button called a granuloma. This is quite harmless but it may need removing, so it's worth getting your GP to have a look.

Colic

This is the name given to the repeated episodes of unsoothable crying that around 20 per cent of normal, healthy babies can have up until they are three months old. During an attack babies usually go red in the face, become rigid and pull their knees up into their tummies. It most often occurs in the evenings and each attack can last for up to a few hours.

It is believed that abdominal pain is to blame for colic, although this has not been proven. In fact, no-one really knows why it occurs.

Unfortunately there's no cure for it either, but there are a number of measures that may help:

- Give your baby colic drops or gripe water – these are available from your local pharmacy.
- Make sure you wind your baby thoroughly after feeds.
- Carry your baby in a sling.
- Rub your baby on its back or tummy.
- If your baby is bottle fed, changing from cow's milk to soya milk seems to help some babies, although there's no proof or scientific reason why this is so.
- If you are breastfeeding, see if there are particular foods in your own diet (curries or chillies, for example) that seem to make your baby's colic worse, then make a point of avoiding them.
- If all else fails, some parents resort to taking their babies out for a drive in the car. While this can settle them temporarily, beware that once you get them out of the car, the symptoms can start all over again.

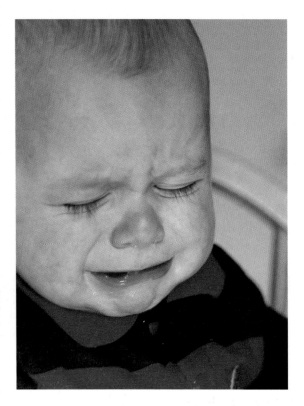

Crying

All babies cry, and this is because they have no other way to attract your attention and they inherently know that this method is particularly foolproof! The amount a baby cries will vary, but you can be sure it will be triggered off by one of a variety of factors, including:

- Hunger.
- Loneliness.
- Boredom.
- Separation.
- Dirty or sodden nappy.
- Colic.
- Pain – nappy rash, wind, etc.

A number of tricks can help to soothe them, such as rocking, a trip in their pram, frequent feeding, rubbing or massage, music, a change of room or environment, or a drive in the car. And, of course, a simple cuddle and the consoling sound of your voice can also work wonders.

If your baby seems inconsolable in their cry and it sounds different to normal, it may be because he or she is unwell, in which case a visit to the doctor would be advisable.

The square mouth

Believe it or not, the first person to give a scientific description of a baby crying was the naturalist and discoverer of the theory of evolution, Charles Darwin, in 1872. 'Infants, when suffering even slight pain or discomfort, utter violent and prolonged screams,' he said, ' ... their eyes are firmly closed, so that the skin round them is wrinkled, and the forehead contracted into a frown. The mouth is widely opened with the lips retracted in a peculiar manner, which causes it to assume a squarish form.'

Sleep

In the first few months of parenthood you probably won't get a lot of shut-eye, because although babies sleep for around eight hours per night, it won't necessarily happen in one go as they are likely to wake frequently for feeds throughout the night (more often if they're breastfed).

One way to combat the problem of broken sleep is to try to get your baby into some kind of bedtime routine – such as bath, story, then bed – as soon as you can, so that they quickly learn the difference between night and day.

Help baby to sleep at night

◊ Always put your baby to sleep in their cot, day or night, so that this place soon becomes associated with bedtime.

◊ You may want to try a dummy, but as we learned with two of ours, when it falls out and they can't find it, they will call you to put it back.

◊ Use a dimmer light during nocturnal visits to avoid over-stimulating them.

◊ Don't change their nappies when they wake for a feed.

◊ When they wake, don't pick them up every time or they'll start waking just for a cuddle. Stroke their heads, say 'night night' and leave them. And certainly don't take them down to the TV room with you.

Your health visitor will have lots more advice about sleep if you run into trouble, or there are many books around to guide you through various sleep-training techniques. If prolonged broken nights really start to get you down, there are a number of specialist clinics around who can help. (See Useful Addresses on page 220.)

Sudden Infant Death Syndrome (SIDS or Cot Death)

Sudden Infant Death Syndrome is the sudden and unexpected death of a baby who is less than one year old, and in whom no obvious cause of death can be found. No-one really knows why this happens, but loads of research has been done to come up with things that can be done to prevent it and minimize the risks, which has resulted in a 75 per cent reduction in the rate of these deaths occuring since 1991.

Tragically, over 300 babies a year still die in the UK as a result of SIDS, most of whom are less than four months old. But you can dramatically reduce the risk of this by following the recommended guidelines from the Department of Health and the Foundation for Sudden Infant Death:

- Always place your baby on their back to sleep; they are nine times more likely to suffer a cot death if they sleep on their fronts than on their backs. However, it's fine (and recommended for their development) to let them play on their fronts as long as you are keeping a good eye on them.

- Cut out smoking in pregnancy (and that includes expectant fathers too) and don't let anyone smoke in the same room as your baby.

- Do not let your baby get too hot (or too cold). A room temperature of around 18°C is just about right, and if your baby feels to you like they are hot in bed, it's OK to take off some of their covers. Use lightweight blankets and put them to sleep with their feet at the foot of the cot so that they don't wriggle underneath the covers. Even in winter, babies who are unwell and feverish need fewer clothes and bedclothes than you would assume. Babies should never sleep with a hot water bottle or electric blanket, or next to a radiator, heater or fire, or in direct sunshine (including when in the car). When it's warm, cool their room by closing the curtains and opening the windows during the day.

- Remove their hats and extra clothing as soon as you get indoors or get on a warm bus or train, or go into a shop, even if it means waking your baby.

- Give them plenty to drink, and in very hot weather you can sponge them down regularly with tepid water.

- Do not share a bed with your baby if you or your partner have been drinking alcohol or have taken drugs, if you are smokers, if your baby was born prematurely, if they are under three months old or if you are excessively tired. The main reasons for this are that you might roll over in your sleep and suffocate them, your baby could get caught between the wall and the bed, or they could simply roll out of your bed and injure themselves. The safest place for your baby to sleep for the first six months is in a cot in your bedroom. And don't fall asleep with them on the sofa either, as this is known to account for 10 per cent of SIDS deaths.

- If your baby is unwell, seek medical advice promptly.

For further advice, visit www.fsid.org.uk

And finally...

After a while you'll get the hang of this parenting lark, the sleep deprivation will be over and your new addition will be a little dream. It's hard to explain the excitement of watching them grow, but each new milestone is amazing to see: their first smile, the day they first sit up, or crawl, or stand to cruise around your furniture. And the day they utter those immortal words 'Mummy' or 'Daddy' for the first time will just blow you away.

It's at times like that when you realize it was all worth it, and the broken nights and sore nipples will pale into insignificance. Of course, it's not always going to be plain sailing bringing up a child, but the positives by far outweigh the negatives. Your life will change beyond recognition, but hopefully for the better.

And when your own parents tell you that you should cherish every moment with your children because they grow up so fast, believe them. Before you know it they'll be independent, potty trained and yakking away at you ten to the dozen. They'll have their own little friends and social lives and be up to all sorts of mischief.

At which point you may start to yearn for the days when they were smaller, when they stayed where you left them and they couldn't answer back. But who knows, it may then be the time for you to start thinking about making another baby. If so, I'd like to refer you back to Chapter 1…

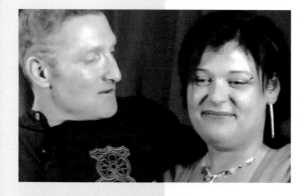

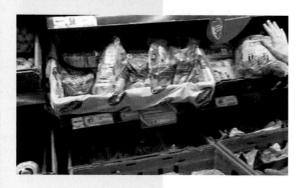

Lifestyle

We know about the importance of trying to keep yourself fit if you want to maximize your chances of conceiving, and how beneficial cutting out fags and booze can be alongside a healthy, well-balanced diet. For Paula and Gary their lifestyles were not just going to be a small hurdle to clear in order to have a baby, but more like a huge mountain to climb. Paula already had an 11-year-old child from a previous relationship but she really wanted a baby with Gary, who she'd been with for four years.

However, both Paula and Gary were smokers and had appalling diets – which could make the task of conceiving quite a struggle. In fact, although Paula smoked 20 to 30 roll ups a day for a while, she had agreed to significantly cut back. Stopping altogether while trying for a baby was unlikely, though, as she was convinced that, 'you need a fag in the morning'. Gary too had a heavy smoking habit; puffing his way through around 20 each day.

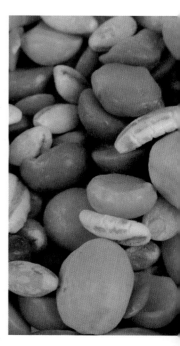

As far as food was concerned, junk was on the menu most days with processed foods, crisps and pastries making up their staple diet. Paula also skipped breakfast (which is a mistake if you want to get your metabolism going each day) in the vain hope that it would help her to lose weight. She did, however, get regular exercise at the gym, dragging Gary along with her around five times per week. Despite the exercise, though, her unhealthy diet meant she was stuck with a BMI of 31.

Although Gary had a fantastic sperm count, their lifestyle could have held them back from conceiving. But by reducing their alcohol and cigarette intake and improving their diet, they soon became pregnant.

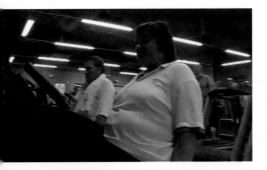

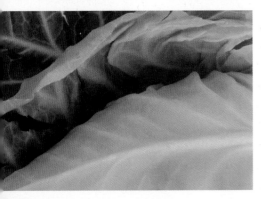

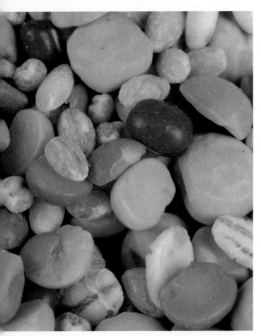

As for sex, the couple were trying to maximize their chances by doing it every day. Gary, however, had a secret weapon to combat the detrimental effects of their lifestyle: he was Mr Supersperm. His count was over 400 million per millilitre – which is way above the desired 20 million per millilitre thought to be needed to conceive.

Despite this breeding advantage they didn't rest on their reproductive laurels and they tried to address their diet and cigarette intake and Paula also lost weight. Their hard work was rewarded when they conceived in November 2005.

At 28 weeks they paid for a private 4-D scan to make sure all was well with the baby. These scans are available at a number of clinics and use high-quality ultrasound technology to allow parents to see a 3-D image of their baby (in which they can see the details of their facial features while still in the womb) and also to pick up all their movements. This means seeing the baby kicking, swimming, smiling, swallowing, sucking its thumb and even yawning.

After a straightforward pregnancy during which she gave up smoking, Paula then gave birth to Sydnee in July 2006.

Case study

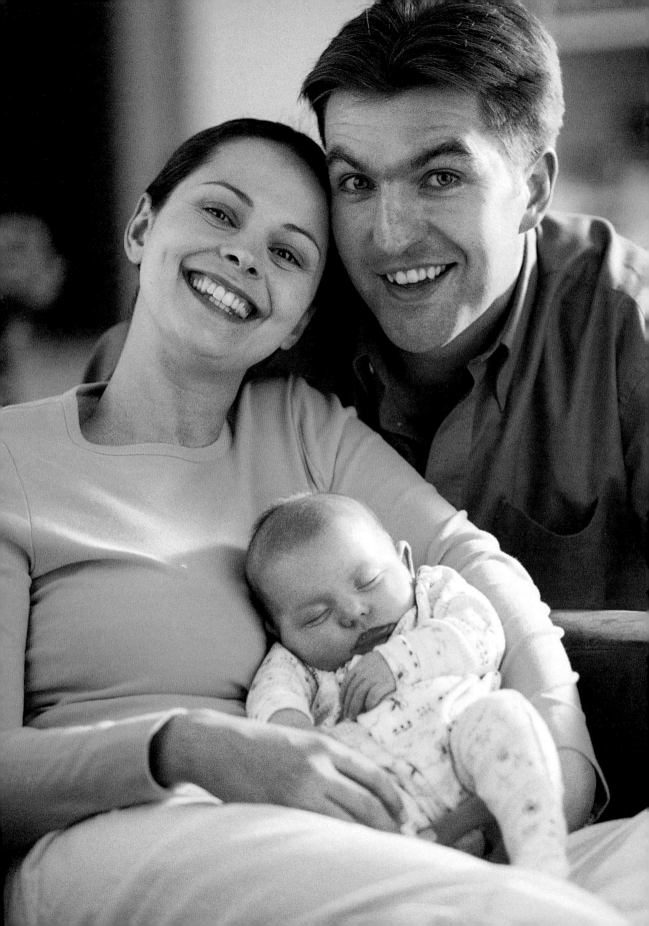

chapter 7

And dad makes three

t's a funny old game being a dad. You're obviously a vital part of the baby-making procedure itself, with an equal share of the conception process, but from the moment the deed is done and you roll apart and start snoring, that's about it from you. The rest of pregnancy is pretty much her business – and for nine months your child is more strictly speaking her child. She grows the baby, feels it enlarging and kicking inside her, and she also gets the sickness, stretch marks and the fun of going through labour, of course.

Where does 'dad' fit in to all this?

There isn't much you can do directly to affect the way your baby will turn out at this point, and consequently many blokes start to feel at best redundant and at worst, indifferent about the whole pregnancy thing.

In fact, probably as a result of this enforced detachment, men have historically absented themselves from pretty much the whole process. Having babies was, by default, women's work; and as for the labour bit, the most some dads would do was pace up and down outside the delivery room until the midwife gave them the nod that their offspring had arrived so that they could scarper down the pub and wet the baby's head.

We're a little bit more enlightened these days, and being a hands-on dad has even become quite cool, with countless 'A' list celebrities happy (some might say desperate) to be seen parading their sprogs around the trendiest stores and eateries, or kicking a ball around with them in the park. As a result, men are much more willing to do their bit in the delivery suite by performing such supportive acts as allowing their hands to be squeezed (often to a degree just short of where fingers are snapped), mopping their partner's brows and even giving encouragement when it's needed!

Yet despite this new attitude of involvement, watching your partner go through the pain of childbirth with the coaching of a midwife (who's usually another woman) still makes most men feel completely helpless. Especially when their other halves dump the blame for all of this pain firmly on their doorsteps (often accompanied by some choice words that have never before passed their lips).

So should we chaps just wait until some bright spark works out a way for us to carry a baby before we take a more active role in pregnancy (and I'm guessing the queue of volunteers for that will be a short one), or can we actually play a useful role already?

Begin at the beginning

The answer to this is yes, of course we can be of help, and if dads are serious about their role in parenthood then they need to get involved at the very start of this amazing journey.

Work with your partner

You've started down this road together, so try to stay together on it. The key to this is not to get left out by getting left behind.

Pregnancy has a whole vocabulary of its own that can end up a secret language between your partner and her female friends if you don't make an effort to learn it. Reading books like this can help you to understand the terminology and keep up with the lingo.

Do your research and find out what's happening to her and how the baby is developing. There are plenty of books, professionals and friends who've been there before and can (and will) give you advice from their knowledge and experience, but this pregnancy is unique to the two of you and as a couple you need to approach it in the way that works best for you.

The best way to come to a mutually agreed plan of action for the next nine months is to talk to each other. Ask your partner about how she's feeling and how she thinks you can help her – whether it's doing some washing or cleaning now and as she gets bigger (when lugging the Hoover around becomes a gargantuan effort), by putting up shelves in the baby's room, or just by taking responsibility for researching which baby monitor or car seat to buy.

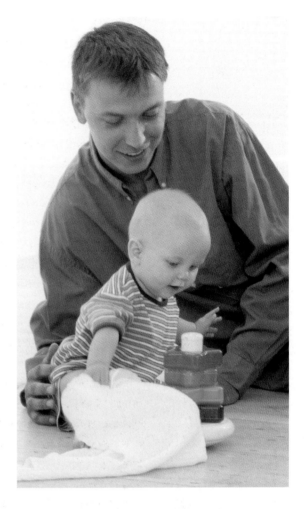

As your partner gets further on into her pregnancy, she will appreciate all the help you can offer.

As she goes through the various stages of pregnancy, your partner may well need a bit of pampering and sympathy – particularly when she's feeling sick/tired/heavy – but don't leave that to her girlfriends, or you'll find yourself feeling even more excluded. Support her through her symptoms and try to be empathetic: the last thing she needs to be told when she's feeling as large and sluggish as an elephant is that she looks like one too.

A crucial part of being in this together is making sure that your relationship doesn't suffer and that you make time to be together, and perhaps even to spend time NOT talking about the baby. This time just as a couple is important and will prove invaluable when supporting one another through the trials and tribulations of parenting over the years ahead; so enjoy it and make it count. Be reassured, too, that it's quite safe to have sex during pregnancy. You will not hurt your baby and it certainly won't (as one male patient of mine thought) make the baby come out with a bruise on its forehead.

Preparing for the new addition

Go with your partner to some of her antenatal appointments and listen to the midwife as she explains about the development of your baby. It is an amazing experience hearing your baby's heartbeat for the first time, and even more amazing actually to see it on a scan. In his book *The Sixty Minute Father,* Rob Parson reminds dads how no-one on their deathbed has said, 'I wish I'd spent more time at the office.' That holds true just as much in the antenatal period as it does after the child is born.

Parenting is a once in a lifetime opportunity – don't miss it.

A major part of preparing for the new arrival at this stage is preparing for its literal arrival. Go along to antenatal classes with your partner, wherever your participation is invited. You're not being wet by learning how to help her breathe in the delivery suite or how to change nappies and bath your baby – they're all vital skills to have if you're going to be a hands-on father.

> Antenatal classes will not only give you all the information you want about the birth and early days with your baby (and probably more details that you wish you hadn't heard), but they will also give you a chance to meet other men who are in the same boat. Chances are they'll be worried about the whole process too, and you can all learn from each others' experiences. Use them as your support network just as your partner might their partners – go for a beer with them now and after the birth, and swap stories and/or concerns that you don't want to worry your partner with.

Don't put off preparing the nursery until the last minute if your partner is nagging you to get on with it. Many women experience nesting urges and you will only increase her stress if the nursery is still full of junk a week before the due date. And you'll certainly hear all about it from her and concerned relatives if she gets on and does the job herself. (Although climbing on and off a step-ladder to paint the ceiling of the nursery did kick-start one of my wife's labours, so when your partner's 40 weeks and flagging you might use that as an incentive for getting some help!)

As the last few weeks count down to the big day, make it your responsibility to ensure that the car is always full of petrol – just in case. Also make sure you're fully versed as to how to fit the car seat and have done a dry run to the hospital – or have at least looked it up on a map – so you know where you're going when it all kicks off.

If possible, try not to book in too many after-work drinks in the final days leading up to the due date – or earlier if you can bear it – and make sure you keep your quota down to a safe level so that you could still drive and be supportive should the baby decide to turn up early. As I mentioned in Chapter 5, I fell into this trap when we were expecting our first and my contracting wife had to drive us both into hospital. I wasn't popular!

When your partner starts packing her bag, make sure you add a change of clothes for yourself. If you get called away from work and have to meet her at the hospital, you might prefer not to spend the labour time in your suit or whatever. If you're unlucky and are in the hospital for the long haul, you might need a change of clothes from one day into the next. Your shirt may also get a battering from the blood and various bodily fluids splashing around in the delivery room, and the last thing you want to do is have to head home looking like you've just stepped out of a war zone.

It's never too soon to talk to your partner and to your work about parental leave. Decide when and how much time you want to take off. If the mother-in-law is ready to swoop in and take control, it might be more beneficial to take time off later when she's gone. Or if, at a later date, you discover that an elective Caesarean is on the cards, you might need to consider carefully who, if not you, can be around to help for the first six weeks until she can drive and pick up the baby with ease.

PATERNITY LEAVE

Under the Employment Act of 2002 fathers are entitled to two weeks' paid paternity leave on top of 13 unpaid weeks' parental leave. It's paid at the same rate as Statutory Maternity Pay and your employer can reclaim it from the government.

To receive this you must have completed 26 weeks of qualifying service with the same employer by the 26th week of pregnancy. Partners or husbands of the mother qualify for paternity leave, but you don't have to be the biological father.

Leave must be taken in a single block of either one week or two weeks, rather than as sporadic days off, and it can be taken any time during the first 56 days after the birth of a child or their expected date of delivery (depending on which is the earliest). This leave is also available to adoptive fathers.

You are entitled to return to the same job following paternity leave and will be protected from unfair dismissal related to paternity leave.

The big day

This is the time that your partner most needs you to be strong and positive – whatever happens. Be there at the birth to support and encourage (and to shut up when need be). You'll never get a better chance to build a special bond with your partner or child.

Talk to your partner about her birthplan before the big day, and make sure you know what she really doesn't want to happen to her, what pain relief she won't consider and, if things don't go according to plan, what she might compromize on in the heat of the moment. You might be called upon to be her voice, so it is important that you know her wishes and get it right in the delivery room to save trouble later!

In the same breath, read up about labour before the big day if you didn't get everything you wanted to know from antenatal classes, and if you're not squeamish. This knowledge will stand you in good stead if your partner is really having a tough time and the doctor wants your consent to perform a forceps or Caesarean delivery.

Be warned, too, that you might be asked by the midwife if you want to cut the cord when the baby is delivered – it's not compulsory, and they won't make you fry it up for breakfast, but the option's there if you want to be literally 'hands-on'.

Coming home

If you haven't proved your love and support by now, then this is the time that all your resources need to be at the ready. Coming home is when your partner (and child) will probably need you the most.

If you've left your partner in hospital after the birth of your child, do by all means go off and tell the world your news and have a celebratory drink, but don't get so trollied you forget to pick your family up in the morning or are so hung over that the first nappy at home sends you running to the bathroom. She may well have not had any sleep the first night either, but for very different reasons – and she won't appreciate it if you are as much use as a chocolate teapot.

Get that caveman instinct going and fend off visitors for the first few days – either at home or at the hospital. Talk to your partner and find out whether you are both happy to receive people. If you are, make sure they don't outstay their welcome or move in against your wishes. You don't have to see everyone in the first week – the novelty of a new baby doesn't wear off that quickly! But

Don't be squeamish about changing nappies – use it as a bonding experience with your baby.

the novelty of having a houseful of people every day when you're both feeling knackered certainly will.

If your partner is breastfeeding then you might feel a bit redundant, but there are still nappies to change and the baby will need bathing. These are ideal father and child bonding sessions, so use them to their full advantage. If you decide to bottle-feed, take the opportunity to feed the baby and have special time with him or her, and to give your partner a break – particularly if she wants to get to bed early before the first night feed and you're happy to stay up and watch *Match of the Day*.

Try to help out as much as you can. If you don't know where to start, then ask her what needs doing – whether it's popping down to the shops for more nappies or food, ordering a take away for dinner, or putting a load of washing on. As blokes our lack of multi-tasking ability is legendary, but if you can get in touch with your more organized, feminine side and even go as far as looking for jobs that need doing before you're asked, you'll go a long way to making her life easier. (Not to mention making you the best husband – as well as the best father – around.)

Push the baby out in the pram, or take him or her out in a sling, whenever you fancy a walk or are popping out to the shops, and give your partner time to recover and catch her breath. A new baby is all-consuming and everyone needs a break.

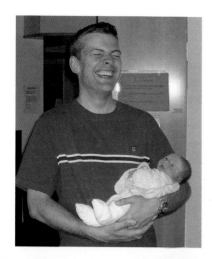

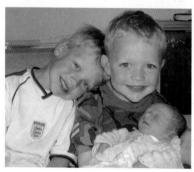

Some priceless moments from my own experiences of fatherhood with Harry, Sam and Archie.

As long as your partner is confident that you won't give the child some ridiculous name, make it your job to go and register the baby. This has to be done within the first 42 days of their birth, and once you've done this you can start claiming your Child Benefit Allowance – so there's an incentive!

There's no doubt that your life changes dramatically when you become a dad – and for some men there can be a big psychological battle between taking on the responsibility of this new role and the desire to be out boozing with the lads like they used to. But the benefits that come with being a father are well worth the aggro, and I for one wouldn't have missed any of it for the world.

Sure, you're torn between the bright lights and late nights of your old life (although parenthood doesn't have to stop you going out and enjoying yourself) and the world of changing nappies and playing boo. But you'll know you've made the transition from lad to dad when: you can sit through countless episodes of *Thomas the Tank Engine* at six in the morning without wanting to stick a fork in your leg to prove you've not slipped into a coma; you turn down tickets to a football match to kick a ball around in the park with your toddler; you find yourself saying 'flubberdubber dub' out loud, not because you've had a skinful but because you're pretending to be a Flowerpot Man to get a smile out of your little one; and when you can catch a handful of half-chewed, half-slobbered on, unrecognizable goo without retching.

But the final proof of your elevated status comes when you can instinctively reach out to wipe the green, sticky snot from your child's nose without losing eye contact with, or breaking conversation with, another adult.

Fatherhood is many things: it's frustrating, tiring, challenging, a test of patience, a test of your resourcefulness, inconvenient, and at times it pushes you to the end of your tether. But it's also motivating, great fun, exciting, exhilarating, varied, has unbelievably happy times and provides wonderful moments that life without children just can't compete with. So it's thoroughly unmissable.

Some blokes never get the chance to experience fatherhood and would give their right arm to be able to – so enjoy it, it's a real privilege.

Useful addresses

Pregnancy and birth

The Active Birth Centre
Bickerton House
25 Bickerton Road
London N19 5JT
020 7281 6760
www.activebirthcentre.com
Classes and information on natural birth and parenting techniques, including prenatal and postnatal yoga and holistic treatments. Online shop for birth and beyond essentials, also for birthing pool hire and sales.

DF Research
12 Smithfield Street
London
EC1A 9LA
Tel: 020 7332 8800
www.drfoster.co.uk/localservices/birthGuide.asp
Offers impartial advice on all maternity units in hospitals in the UK.

The Centre for Reproductive Medicine
4 Priory Road
Clifton
Bristol BS8 1TY
0117 902 1100
www.repromed.co.uk
Provides information on infertility, IVF and NHS provision.

La Leche League (Great Britain)
PO Box 29
West Bridgford
Nottingham NG2 7NP
Breastfeeding line: 0845 120 2918
www.laleche.org.uk
Advice and support for mothers on breastfeeding.

National Childbirth Trust
Alexandra House
Oldham Terrace
Acton
London W3 6NH
Enquiry Line: 0870 444 8707
www.nct.org.uk
Branches across the country offer local antenatal classes, social events, clothes and accessories sales and postnatal and breastfeeding advice and support.

NHS Direct
08454647
www.nhsdirect.nhs.uk
24-hour advice about symptoms in pregnancy and health needs of young children.

Support

The Association for Postnatal Illness
145 Dawes Road
London SW6 7EB
020 7386 0868
www.apni.org
Provides support for mothers suffering from post-natal illness.

BLISS (Baby Life Support Systems)
2nd and 3rd Floors
9 Holyrood Street
London Bridge
London SE1 2EL
020 7378 1122
helpline: Freephone 0500 618140
www.bliss.org.uk
Support for parents and families of premature and special care babies.

Cry-sis
BM Cry-sis
London WC1N 3XX
08451 228 669
www.cry-sis.org.uk
Offers support and advice for families with excessively crying, sleepless and demanding babies.

Gingerbread
307 Borough High Street
London SE1 1JH
020 7403 9500
www.gingerbread.org.uk
Support organisation for one-parent families offering advice through a helpline and local self-help groups.

Millpond Sleep Clinic
020 8444 0040
www.mill-pond.co.uk
Private clinic offering advice for families experiencing baby and child sleep problems.

The Miscarriage Association
c/o Clayton Hospital
Northgate
Wakefield
West Yorkshire WF1 3JS
helpline: 01924 200799
www.miscarriageassociation.org.uk
Advice and support for those who have suffered a miscarriage.

Multiple Births Foundation
Hammersmith House Level 4
Queen Charlotte's & Chelsea Hospital
Du Cane Road
London, W12 0HS
020 8383 3519
www.multiplebirths.org.uk
Works to improve the care and support of multiple birth families.

One Parent Families
255 Kentish Town Road
London NW5 2LX
020 7428 5400
www.oneparentfamilies.org.uk
Helpline: 0800 018 5026
Offers information on childcare, tax credits, benefits and local groups for one parent families.

Children with special needs

Association for Spina Bifida and Hydrocephalus (ASBAH)

Asbah House
42 Park Road
Peterborough
Cambridgeshire PE1 2UQ
01733 555988
Helpline: 0845 450 7755
www.asbah.org
Provides advice and information for parents and carers of children with spina bifida and hydrocephalus.

Down's Syndrome Association

Langdon Down Centre
2a Langdon Park
Teddington
TW11 9PS
0845 230 0372
www.downs-syndrome.org.uk
Helpline and support for people with Down's syndrome and their families.

MENCAP

123 Golden Lane
London EC1Y 0RT
England: 020 7545 0454
Northern Ireland: 02890 691351
Wales: 02920 747588
www.mencap.org.uk
Support and advice for families of children with learning difficulties.

Scope

6 Market Road
London N7 9PW
0800 800 3333
www.scope.org.uk
Information and help for people with cerebral palsy and their parents and carers.

Family planning

British Pregnancy Advisory Service (BPAS)

4th Floor

Amec House

Timothy's Bridge Road

Stratford-upon-Avon CV37 9BF

08457 30 40 30

www.bpas.org

Advice on contraception.

Brook

421 Highgate Studios

53-79 Highgate Road

London NW5 1TL

020 7284 6040

www.brook.org.uk

Charity that offers centres throughout Britain which provide free and confidential professional sexual health, contraception and pregnancy advice for people under 25 years old.

The Family Planning Association

50 Featherstone Street

London EC1Y 8QU

Helpline: 0845 310 1334

www.fpa.org.uk

Information about family planning and sexual health.

Marie Stopes International

153-157 Cleveland Street

London W1T 6QW

0845 300 80 90

www.mariestopes.org.uk

Information about sexual and reproductive health.

Acknowledgements

Firstly I would like to thank the production team at Mentorn Television for not only giving me the chance to present the series *Make Me a Baby* and therefore to be offered the opportunity to write this book, but also for making my virginal television experience such a pleasurable one. Particular thanks go to: Liesel Evans, Jennifer Gilroy, Arlene Jeffrey and Jane Rogerson.

Thanks too to the excellent editorial team at BBC Active, to Emma Shackleton for having enough faith to commission me to write this book and to Helena Caldon for her hard work, enthusiasm, advice, encouragement and for the many polite ways she developed to help keep me on track. I'd also like to thank Annette Peppis for the work she did on the fantastic design.

I am also indebted to my friends and colleagues at the Fishponds Family Practice, for their encouragement while completing this project and for making it easy to take time out to complete it.

My wife Nikki needs special thanks for putting up with my absences both while filming and writing and for so much more.

This book is dedicated to the memory of my Dad and to my Mum, without whom… And to Harry, Sam and Archie, the three babies that I helped to make.

Couples who participated in *Make Me a Baby*

Abigail & Andrew Catlender
Adele & Jim Stevenson
Adrianna & Jonathan Kelly
Aneluta & Philip Hurwood
Angela & Odaatei Nanka-Bruce
Anita Foss & Paul Line
Anne Newbery & Paul Bland
Annette & Daniel Jones
Annette & Ian Hall
Ashley & Faye Moreton-Barker
Barbara & Andy Benner
Becky & Jobi Hold
Bex & Will Cambridge
Caroline & Peter Jones
Chantelle Brown & Kyle James
Charlotte & Simon Townsend
Clair & Lyndon Rivers Boyden
Claire & Anthony Sherrick
Claire & Darren Thompson
Claudia & Matthew Nock-Fuerst
Dalia Alsawy & Osama Shaheen

Dean & Louise Woods
Elisabeth Taylor & Chris Taylor
Ellen & Matt Sweeney
Ellen Louise Firbank & James Lockhart
Emma Frost & John Dixon
Eve & Damian Stone
Faye & Michael Bell
Gail & Gordon Meadow
Gezina & Eugene Marais
Hannah & David Skelly
Hannah & Marvin Tress
Helen & John Bullas
Helen Braid & Martin Feasey
Jackie & Stephen Barr
Jane & Simon Thurman
Jill and Andrew Cox
Johanne & Stuart Gillott
Jude & Gary Robinson
Julia Madden & Osivaldo Rodriguez
Juliet & Paul Wilder
Karen & Ben Brown

Karen & James Rogers
Karen & Steven Muir
Kate & Pete Goodhead
Kate Wheeler & Glenn Lockey
Kellie Campbell & Andy Webb
Kelly Hearne & Alec Carmichael
Kim & Jamie Wadman
Kim & John White
Laura Blackburn Finlay & Magnus Finlay
Leanne & Craig Cooper
Leeann & Danny Demarzo
Lewis Jam & Jovia Nabukwasi
Louisa Morris & Sean Davies
Louise & David Morgon
Lucinda Hitchcock & Anthony Carder
Lyn & Jonathan Blackham
Lyndsey Hay & Kevin Shaw
May & Paul Edmundson
Melodie & Mark Evans
Michele & Joseph Chiemeka
Michelle & Graeme Brighten

Natasha & Stuart Kearney
Neil & Kate Gregory
Pamela Graham & Ian Buers
Patsy Reynolds & Michael Robb
Paula Ives & Gary Dean
Paula Smith & Kevin Malone
Philipa Stratford & Simon Marsh
Rachael Paylor & Mark Green
Rachel & Keith Duffield
Rachel & Martin Murphy
Rhiannon & Sergiy Zhuravlyova
Ruth & Jonathan Killow
Sam & Scott Muter

Sam Rivers & Chris Gofton
Sandra Harkness & Colin Greenaway
Sarah & Colin Yates
Sarah & Graham Revers-Jackson
Sarah & Richard Iles
Sarah & Stuart Neil
Sarah Darch & Ivan Darch
Sarah Ellis-Randall & Jody Randall
Selina Nylander & Des Nylander
Shanelle Jordaan & Francois Moizant
Sharon Nicholl & Raymond Seel
Stephanie & Richard Metson
Sue & Craig Hillbeck

Susan & Allan Jackson
Susan & Jon Bryant
Susan Holtham & Alan Koeninger
Suzanne & Christian Hubble
Suzannel & Charles Linskaill
Tina & Peter Rose
Tracy & John McCormack
Trudi & Mark Penny
Valerie & Thomas Liebers
Victoria Driscoll & Les Ayaoge
Yvette Mahon & Andrew Farrer

Picture credits